Advance Praise for
THE NEW WOMAN'S GUIDE
TO HEALTHY AGING

"As a long-time patient of Dr. Brown, I was delighted to endorse the first edition of her book. Now I am even more pleased to recommend this second edition, with its important revisions and a brand-new chapter on women's sexual health. As a doctor, Vivien Brown's advice is solid and practical; as a woman, her guidance is specialized and appreciated. I sincerely hope you will seize the opportunity to learn and benefit from her insightful approach to wellness and aging."

—Kirstine Stewart, media and tech executive and author

"Having worked with Dr. Vivien Brown for the better part of 40 years, I never cease to be amazed by her ability to teach and explain medical issues in a way that everyone can understand. The complex becomes clarified, and the knowledge she delivers becomes a powerful tool for all of us to channel so that we can become healthier."

—Sheldon Elman, MD, founder and chairman emeritus, Medisys; chairman, Esplanade Ventures; executive chairman, Carebook

"As a cofounder of one of Canada's foremost training and education enterprises in the medical field, and as a former teacher, I know the passion that drives someone to want to share knowledge. Dr. Vivien Brown exemplifies this passion in her medical practice, in her international speaking engagements, in her life. She has made it her mission, as a doctor and as a woman, to spread this knowledge as widely as possible. This book goes a long way toward achieving that goal. Highly recommended for anyone who wants to stay on top of the latest in health advances for women."

—Susan Caldwell, founder and strat

THE NEW WOMAN'S GUIDE TO HEALTHY AGING

*Eight Proven Ways
to Keep You Vibrant,
Happy & Strong*

Vivien Brown, M.D.

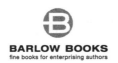

BARLOW BOOKS
fine books for enterprising authors

Library and Archives Canada Cataloguing in Publication data available upon request.

ISBN 978-1-988025-62-9 (paperback)

Printed in Canada

Publisher: Sarah Scott
Cover photograph: Lorella Zanetti
Marketing & publicity: Debby de Groot

For more information, visit www.barlowbooks.com.

Barlow Book Publishing Inc.
96 Elm Avenue, Toronto, ON
Canada M4W 1P2

BARLOW
BOOKS

For Rivy and
Murray Perelman

My mother was a courageous woman
and an incredible role model, and my
father was a feminist long before it was
fashionable to be one. They instilled
in me the confidence to succeed, and
I am forever grateful. This edition is
dedicated to their memory.

Contents

Foreword

With this edition of *The NEW Woman's Guide to Healthy Aging*, Dr. Vivien Brown contributes a much-needed addition to the canon of popular medical literature—advice for women on how to do their part to ensure they age as healthfully and vitally as possible, both physically and cognitively. A great communicator and an accomplished physician, Dr. Brown makes sometimes-complicated medical issues clear and understandable. This ability to bring a human voice to scientific and medical data has made her an invaluable resource on the board of Women's Brain Health Initiative since its creation in 2012.

The pace of medical research in the modern world is truly astounding; new discoveries and new understandings seem to come almost daily. It is nearly impossible for most people outside the medical community to keep current, and it is often difficult to understand important new medical recommendations that emerge.

Thankfully, it is part of your physician's responsibility to keep abreast of the latest research and to explain the conclusions of that research so that you understand the reasons for your doctor's advice. To that end, Dr. Brown has revised the content of many chapters based on the latest research, and she presents the information in a direct and practical way.

With the inclusion in this edition of a new chapter on women's sexual health, Dr. Brown discusses eight important areas of women's health. Her aim is to give you the information you need to become your own best health advocate and a partner with your physician in your medical care. With this book, she succeeds admirably in achieving that goal.

Lynn Posluns
Founder and President, Women's Brain Health Initiative

Preface

Welcome to *The NEW Woman's Guide to Healthy Aging: Eight Proven Ways to Keep You Vibrant, Happy, & Strong.* If you are like me, you want to remain sound in body and mind well into old age. For most of us, a healthy old age is our final destination. And as with every destination, it involves a journey.

Oliver Wendell Holmes once said, "I find the great thing in this world is not so much where we stand, as in what direction we are moving." That quotation expresses an underlying theme of this book: it is never too early, or too late, to start moving in the direction of a vital and independent old age.

Perhaps in your journey through life you have always been on the path to a healthy old age—you've made lifestyle choices that enhance your chances of avoiding physical diseases and cognitive impairment. Perhaps you are just stepping onto that path for the first time—you've recently realized that it's time to change some potentially damaging habits. Or perhaps you remain reluctant to take that first step—you think, "*Que sera, sera*. Whatever will be, will be. So why worry?" Whichever of these descriptions reflects where you are today, my hope is that this book will prove to be a useful guide—a companion—to keep you on the path if you're already on it, to reassure you that your recent decision to follow it is the right decision, to urge you to take that first step if you are still not convinced it's the right path for you.

As with every worthwhile journey, it is not just the destination that matters but also the journey itself. This book is not just about living into your 90s and still being healthy; it is also about enjoying the journey of getting there—it is about a journey that includes the friendships, the motivations, the activities, and the healthy choices you make along the way so that when you do get to 90 you can look back and say, "I feel good about what I did to get here. And I feel good now!"

When I started practising medicine several decades ago, women were undervalued by the medical community in a variety of ways. For example, the model for determining drug dosages for women was very much a male model. When doctors prescribed a medication for a woman, they might consider her "two-thirds of a man," based on average body weights, and therefore prescribe about two-thirds of the dose a man would get. There was little understanding that metabolically women and men are quite different, that drugs do not always work the same way in a woman as they do in a man.

Nor was there much of an appreciation of the fact that a particular health problem might present differently in men and women. We have learned, however, that this is true in cardiac health as well as in brain health. There is also a greater understanding today of how hormones and the state of hormonal balance affect a woman's health. And we now know that women are more prone to certain diseases than are men.

We have learned a lot—are learning a lot—specifically about women's health, but this is not a medical encyclopedia. It is not a treatise. You will not find a thousand technical terms and their definitions. You will not need a dictionary by your side as you read. You will not find footnotes on each page; in fact, you will not find footnotes on any page, although I do acknowledge the contribution of important sources in a separate section at the back of the book.

I see this book as a conversation between you and me, a conversation about your health now, about aging, and about not only maintaining your health as you age but also improving it. As a family doctor I have worked primarily in one-on-one patient care, and women's health has always been a very important focus of my practice. In the past few years I have also taken on a teaching role—teaching new physicians so that they can apply in their own work what my many years of practice have taught me, and teaching in the community so that women become knowledgeable about medical issues that they absolutely *should* be aware of. This book marries what I have learned from my patients and what I have learned as a teacher; it marries information from the latest research with practical steps you can take to apply that information. My hope is that you will learn from it the things you need to know to take control of and enhance your own health.

As a result of COVID-19, there has been a major change in a previously underutilized tool for taking control of and enhancing your health: virtual care (also called telemedicine or telehealth). Because of the pandemic, virtual care has become an important aspect of patient care and is likely to remain so going forward.

Before the pandemic, it was already clear that virtual care was creating a niche for itself in family medicine. Some patients never tried virtual care and some adopted aspects of virtual care readily, but there was no sense of urgency about it. Now, however, COVID-19 has irrevocably altered the health care landscape. With the clear public health directives of staying home, maintaining social distancing, and practising varying degrees of social/physical isolation, virtual care is no longer elective. Rather than being a reasonable option, it is suddenly the absolute norm, the necessity, the first step in accessing medical care.

Family doctors are often thought of as the gatekeepers in health care. With the patient as partner, we evaluate a given condition or concern and decide if a specialty consult is needed, what laboratory tests or types of imaging are required, whether the condition needs treatment, and, if so, what form that treatment should take. A prescription? Physiotherapy? A surgical intervention? What is the next step for the patient?

Because of the potential danger of face-to-face examinations, the COVID-19 experience has taught us the incredible value of virtual care. For example, I have met with patients privately by phone and online. We have discussed issues ranging from elevated levels of cholesterol and the impact on cardiac risk to evaluation of acne, with clear pictures and discussion. We have managed anxiety, urinary infections, early pregnancy questions, and upper respiratory issues. Medication monitoring has been managed virtually, including renewals, changes of dose, the proper duration and intervals of use, and any questions a patient may have had. More than 80 percent of patient visits have been successfully negotiated online. We doctors are still the gatekeepers, but that "gate" now includes deciding whether an in-office visit is necessary.

Of course, not every medical issue can be assessed virtually. Some areas of examination absolutely require in-person consults. But because we have seen that so many different medical issues can be handled equally well in a virtual consult as in an office visit, you should expect virtual care to become a larger part of your physician's normal practice.

So, what does this mean for you? Well, it means it really is time to become more comfortable with using your computer, your e-mail, and your phone as tools to manage your health because there is a good chance your next appointment with your doctor will be online. And the appointment after that, and maybe even the one after that. This is how we will stay connected going forward. This is how we will stay well. This is part of how we will protect our families and ourselves.

You may be asking yourself: will I ever see my doctor again? Of course you will! Virtual care will never replace your physician—it is simply a great new option for communication when an office visit really is not necessary. (See Section C in the Appendix for a ten-step guide to making your virtual medical visit efficient and effective.)

In closing, let me repeat: I hope you will learn from this book the things you need to know to take control of and enhance your health. Medical knowledge is always evolving, and my goal is to keep you up to date with what is new and important in women's health. Here you will find essential recent information about a variety of medical issues that affect your health at every stage of life, and especially as you age. I hope that in addition to digesting the information itself, you will pay careful attention to the language used to describe various conditions. It is language you can use to communicate effectively with your doctor. Clear communication between doctor and patient has always been important, but especially now in our time of increasing virtual care. Having the right vocabulary can help ensure the advice your physician offers is appropriately focused on your specific concerns.

Introduction

*T*he NEW *Woman's Guide to Healthy Aging: Eight Proven Ways to Keep You Vibrant, Happy, & Strong* is all about you as a woman in the early 21st century and your ongoing health as the century continues to unfold. It is about aging well as the years pass by so that you remain vital and independent for as long as possible.

In this book I focus on eight health topics, each in a separate chapter—nutrition, exercise and sleep, brain health, immunization and disease prevention, menopause, cardiac health, osteoporosis, and women's sexual health. There are many more topics I could have included, but I chose these because they are areas that affect almost every woman. Here is a bird's-eye view of what you can expect to find in each chapter.

Chapter 1, The Edible Feast: Diet and Nutrition, is so named because most of us could stand to improve the way we eat.

This chapter discusses the importance of good nutrition throughout life and the harmful impact of poor nutrition on immediate and long-term health. Section A in the Appendix contains information related to this chapter, such as details of Body Mass Index, the MIND diet and dietary recommendations from Health Canada, and additional information about cholesterol and calcium.

Chapter 2, Pump It Up and Let It Rest: Exercise and Sleep, explains why activity and rest are essential to health and what can happen if you do not get enough of either. Section B in the Appendix contains exercise recommendations from Health Canada and links to the exercise recommendations of the Heart and Stroke Foundation of Canada and of Osteoporosis Canada.

Chapter 3, Healthy Hemispheres: The Aging Brain, discusses anatomical and physiological differences between men's brains and women's brains and consequent differences between men and women in brain health.

Chapter 4, The Value of Vaccines: Immunization-Preventable Diseases, includes information about disease prevention and the incredible advances medical science has made in vaccine research and creation. It lists and discusses the vaccines that every healthy woman should be sure to have.

Chapter 5, Marking Middle Age: Menopause and After, covers the impact that loss of estrogen has on a woman's health. It discusses the symptoms of menopause and the sometimes controversial topic of hormone therapy, including how to decide—with your doctor—if it is right for you.

Chapter 6, Happy Valentine's Day: Maintaining Heart Health, explains how a woman's experience of heart disease may differ from a man's and what this means for women's heart health.

Chapter 7, Robust or Brittle? Bone Health and Osteoporosis, discusses exactly what osteoporosis does to bones and explains the first-line treatments for this disease. A photographic illustration in this chapter, comparing healthy bone and osteoporotic bone, proves the old adage, "A picture is worth a thousand words." The chapter also makes the point that osteoporosis is not a normal part of aging and provides strategies to protect your bone health.

Chapter 8, Intimate Differences: Sexuality and Health, discusses the fact that a satisfying sex life is a normal component of good health. It points out, however, that many women experience a lack of sexual interest and desire and that there is a great degree of commonality in their experience. Finally, it highlights two new and effective pharmaceutical options that, according to many women who have used them, can change both attitude and experience for the better.

Thanks to advances in medical science, we now have great options for disease prevention, options that are easy to understand and easy to implement in our daily lives. We also have an abundance of information about strategies to reduce the risk of developing cognitive impairment. Nothing is failsafe: genetic and environmental factors can override even our most valiant efforts to attain and maintain good health. But this book will give you both solid information and practical tools to tilt the odds in your favour and reduce your risk of serious physical and cognitive problems as you age.

In the end, it is up to each of us to do our part to remain vital and healthy. In fact, it is both a personal and a social responsibility. Please be assured: taking time to take care of yourself is selfless, not selfish. Why? Well, among the many things that COVID-19 has taught us is the extent of our inter-connectedness. And that interconnectedness requires us to be proactive. Maintaining our health means maintaining our ability to contribute to the well-being of our families and of our communities, and to have a productive impact on society. As individuals we can do our very best, and with the right health and social policies in place, as a community we can do even better.

But, you know what they say: advice works only if you act on it. I hope you will.

1

THE EDIBLE FEAST

Diet and Nutrition

For many of us, diet is just another four-letter word. Have you ever wondered why the first three letters in it spell "die"? Maybe because that's what we feel like doing when we're in the middle of a weight-loss program. And exercise? Well, I've heard that some people actually enjoy exercising—running, rowing, sweating, swimming, lifting heavy metal plates, or pushing against resistance machines till their muscles ache. They are the lucky ones, I guess, because we all know exercise is good for us, but it seems the majority of people consider anything that resembles strenuous physical activity to be just a little too much work. Sleep, though, we can pretty much all agree on: sometimes it feels like there's nothing quite so wonderful as a good night's sleep ... and nothing quite so horrible as the day after a bad one.

Any way we look at it, though, and regardless of our personal inclinations—whether we're trim or we tip the scale, whether we live to run or we balk at running, whether we sleep like babies or get nothing better than a series of cat-naps through the night—nutrition, exercise, and sleep are among the major factors that affect our health. And one very important thing to realize about these factors is that they are within our control. Sure, other factors beyond our control also affect our health, including family history and genetic inheritance, sex, and age. We cannot modify those, but we can modify how we eat, how active we are, and how well we sleep. And for many of us, some modification is necessary if we want to live a long and healthy life.

In this chapter, let's take a look at some of the problems associated with our modern diet and consider some common-sense solutions that can help reduce your health risk for the long haul. In the next chapter, we will see how a reasonable level of activity and restorative sleep enhance our current well-being and position us for long-term vitality.

"Diet" Does Not Equal "Lose Weight" ... But Some of Us Do Need to Do Just That

One thing I'd like every woman to understand is the true meaning of diet. I cannot emphasize enough how much potential harm comes from our society's insistence that diet simply means restricting caloric intake in order to lose weight.

According to the Canadian Oxford Dictionary, that is included in the *second* definition of diet: "A special course of food to which a person restricts themselves, either to lose weight or for medical reasons." The first meaning of diet is "The kinds of food that a person, animal, or community habitually eats." And it is this first definition that we should all think of when we think of our own diets.

Do you need any proof that the weight-loss definition of diet is widely held? If so, consider this: an estimated 57 percent of American women are currently trying to lose those extra uncomfortable pounds! They are contributing their hard-earned money to the $60 billion spent annually on dieting. But the diet industry aside, why does how we think about the word make any difference?

Here's why. Too many people who think that "diet" equals "lose weight" never take the time to think about the first meaning of diet—that is, the way they eat every day, day in and day out, week in and week out, month after month, when they are *not* trying to lose weight. But from the point of view of healthy living and healthy aging, it is precisely by paying attention to that meaning of diet that we realize the greatest health benefits.

If you're like most women, when you're dieting you're constantly thinking about what you *should* be eating—and also about what you *should not* and *cannot* be eating. To put it another way, you are planning carefully how you eat and maintaining awareness of what you eat. And that is exactly what you should do when you are not dieting. A change in your habits that results in obsession about what you are not eating is not a good change. What I am suggesting is simply that you take the time to understand what healthy eating looks like and do your best to eat that way. If you find you can't do it all the time, try to follow the 80-20 rule.

What is the 80-20 rule when it comes to eating? Simple. It is eating well, eating nutritiously, eating smart 80 percent of the time. And what about the other 20 percent of the time? That's the time you get to indulge in some of your favourite foods, foods that may not actually be that good for you. So when you're at your niece's wedding, go ahead and have that piece of wedding cake, and don't worry about it. You can even have two pieces, but when the wedding reception is over, make sure you get back into that 80 percent zone. Ashley Grachnik, RD, CDE, a Registered Dietitian and Certified Diabetes Educator, is a proponent of the 80-20 rule; she says, though, "It is important to know which foods should make up the 80 percent and which should make up the 20 percent!"

Speaking of your niece's wedding, all too often our concern about weight is really a concern about how we look, not about how fit or healthy we are. It's about trying to look good for that wedding, maybe trying to fit into the dress size you wore when you were the bride's age. (Really? Come on!) But when I talk about adopting a nutritious, healthful diet, that's not what I'm talking about. No; I'm talking about changing the way you think about food—and the way you eat—so that you'll be around for your granddaughter's wedding as well.

Obesity

One result of our failure to think about how we eat is the alarming increase in the rate of obesity in North America over the past several generations. Perhaps we have become too complacent. We have come to accept the notion that life expectancy in North America will continue to rise indefinitely, following its upward trajectory of the past two centuries. The meteoric increase in our standard of living, important advances in medical care and public health, more consistent, year-round access to nutritious foods, and a widespread understanding of what constitutes a healthy lifestyle all contribute to this greater longevity. But based on the increasing obesity rates in North America, the fact is that life expectancy may actually be declining in the 21st century—for the first time in hundreds of years! You have undoubtedly heard the popular mantra "60 is the new 40," and if you have the right combination of genes and lifestyle that may be true for you, but I have concerns that 40 may well be the new 60 as we face the consequences of obesity, diabetes, and lifestyles.

Is there actually an "obesity epidemic," as so many suggest? Let's look at the science to answer that question. A study published in the *New England Journal of Medicine* looked at obesity among American adults and found that obesity rates increased by approximately 50 percent through the 1980s and 1990s after having been relatively stable in the 1960s and 1970s. That was likely the start of it all. An article in the *Journal of the American Medical Association* (April 4, 2016) found that age-adjusted death rates in 2015 increased significantly from the year before; causes of deaths related to obesity were a major factor in the increase. The same article points out that life expectancy in the United States increased consistently between 1961 and 1983, but between 1983 and 1999 life expectancy decreased for men and for women in U.S. counties where obesity was prevalent. The article states that "in addition to the health-related effects, the economic effects of obesity-related disease are substantial and predicted to worsen." So, yes, I think we can conclude that there really is an obesity epidemic. And not just in the United States.

In Canada, approximately 25 percent of adults are obese. Obesity rates for both men and women are about twice as high today as they were in 1981. Along with its growing prevalence, obesity is also becoming more severe, and the research shows that overall fitness levels are decreasing as the incidence of obesity rises. If we include statistics on overweight along with statistics on obesity, we find that 66 percent of Canadian men and 53 percent of Canadian women aged 18 to 79 are overweight or obese, according to Statistics Canada (see URL in Section A of the Appendix).

But what exactly do we mean by obesity? Obesity refers to excessive weight for your height and body frame, based on Body Mass Index (BMI) guidelines. (Section A in the

Appendix explains how to calculate your own BMI.) This is a useful tool, but it has its drawbacks. For instance, it is based on the ratio of a person's weight in kilograms divided by their height in metres squared, but it does not take into account how much of their weight comes from fat and how much from muscle. Because muscle weighs more than fat, people who are muscular may have a higher BMI and still be in excellent health.

If we don't know the fat/muscle breakdown, another—and perhaps even more useful—way to measure obesity is to look at waist circumference. For women, a healthy waist circumference should be no more than 90 centimetres (35 inches). Healthy waist size varies, of course, based on a number of factors, including a woman's height and bone structure, and even ethnicity: as a rule, for Asian women it should be no more than 80 centimetres (31.5 inches).

Waist circumference is a helpful health indicator because it correlates more closely with a number of health risks than either weight or BMI alone. And it turns out that the old apple or pear comparison is accurate. If we look at two women who are the same height and who are equally overweight, and one carries most of the excess weight in her hip area while the other carries it mostly in her protruding belly, we find that the second woman is more at risk than the first not only for heart disease but also for diabetes and other metabolic conditions. Why is this the case? Because the presence of that belly fat indicates that there is fat in and around the organs, fat that can compromise normal organ functioning and lead to liver and kidney problems. So ladies, whatever your weight, it is more important that your waist is smaller and your belly is flatter, even if you end up looking more hippy than you would like. Yes, that does mean you need to exercise to counter the effects of midlife spread, as discussed in the next chapter.

Patients sometime ask me (and it's a reasonable question), "What if I have liposuction to remove some of the fat around my waist—will that help?" The answer is that it may help you look slimmer for a while but it will not improve your health risk because liposuction removes only subcutaneous fat, which is fat that sits right under your skin. Unfortunately, it has no effect at all on intra-abdominal fat, which is the fat that ambushes your organs and squishes all around them and puts you at risk.

On another note, Wallis Simpson, the Duchess of Windsor, is widely credited with saying, "You can never be too rich or too thin." It's catchy, but is it accurate? I am not aware of any research that examines whether a person can be too rich, but there is clear empirical evidence that a person *can* be too thin. I am not simply referring here to research on anorexia, a complicated, life-threatening pathology characterized by a distorted perception of weight. I am also talking about disordered eating: anorexia is an eating disorder, but many women suffer from disordered eating. Disordered eating includes a singular focus on aiming to be thinner than your particular body was naturally designed to be, it includes caloric restriction on an ongoing basis, and it includes excessive exercise.

Being excessively thin can be as harmful to your health as being excessively fat, with negative long-term effects on every body system. Women on the extreme ends of the bell curve—those who weigh too little and those who weigh too much—are at a higher risk of death. Even if the reason for excessive thinness is over-exercising rather than under-eating, it can set a woman up for numerous health issues as she ages. People may say to her all the time, "You look so well," but the truth is that most likely she isn't, or at least that she will not be for long. The message here? Know your body and embrace whatever size you naturally are. You'll be happier—and healthier—if you do.

A Winning Strategy for Losing: Maintaining a Healthy Weight with the *Non-Diet Approach*

The current trend in maintaining a healthy weight is the non-diet approach for health, and although I say trend, it is more than just trendy. It is not like the dozens of fad diets that have had brief popular appeal over the past 50 years. Those diets promise quick weight loss, and they often deliver what they promise—*while* you starve your body in one way or another. But for most dieters, once the dieting ends the pounds soon start reappearing, and many people end up heavier than they were when they started. Sound familiar? Yo-yo dieting (referred to in medical research as *weight cycling*) can be extremely dangerous to your health: for instance, a study by the U.S. National Institutes of Health published in 2015 concluded that "weight cycling was associated with increased diabetes risk, compared with stable weight."

The non-diet approach is a more balanced, realistic way to lose weight and maintain good health with nourishing foods, daily physical activity, positive thinking, and smart lifestyle choices. People who follow it choose a balanced, varied diet rich in whole grains, vegetables, berries, nuts, legumes, fish, poultry, and red wine or grape juice. Yes, you can enjoy your glass of wine and not feel guilty about it!

What does the non-diet approach actually look like? Let's take a look. (See Section A in the Appendix for detailed descriptions of healthy eating regimens, including the MIND diet and links to information about the Mediterranean diet, the DASH diet, and Canada's Food Guide. I also discuss the Mediterranean and MIND diets as they relate to brain health in Chapter 3.)

Non-diet tips for healthy eating

*Avoid portion distortion**

Even if you eat healthy foods, you'll end up gaining unwanted pounds if you consistently eat too much of them. Portion control can be difficult. However, it is easy to do if you know how to balance your plate. The Canadian Diabetes Association recommends using the plate method. Lay your knife across the plate to separate the plate into two halves. Fill one-half up with vegetables. Veggies are loaded with fibre, so they help fill you up; they are low in starch, so they don't raise blood sugars; and they're also low in fat, so no unnecessary calories here. Now use your fork to separate the other half of your plate into quarters. One-quarter is for your starch (one cup of whole-grain pasta, or one small baked potato, or half a cup of brown rice), and the other quarter is for your protein (four to five ounces of meat, fish, or poultry). Still hungry after you've eaten that plateful? Wait about 10 minutes, and if your hunger persists then go back for seconds, but make it seconds of your veggies only … you likely won't still be hungry after that!

Make fibre your friend*

Fibre is a part of plant-based foods that we can't easily digest or absorb into our bloodstream. Fibre keeps our digestive system running smoothly, and it also keeps us feeling full and satisfied longer, so when you add healthy portions of fibre to your diet it's easier to cut back on less healthy foods that contain too much fat, salt, and sugar.

Here is one easy way to boost your fibre: *Be uptight about white*. Choose whole grains instead of highly processed white grains. White bread, white pasta, white rice—these are all

---

*Quoted from the blog of Ashley Grachnik, RD, CDE, Registered Dietitian and Certified Diabetes Educator

processed to the point that very little fibre remains in them. Another way to is choose whole fruit over fruit juice. When is the last time you ate three or four oranges in a sitting? Maybe never? But it takes that many to get the amount of juice in a medium-sized glass. The juice has no fibre and contains a significant amount of sugar; one medium-sized orange, on the other hand, will give you some fibre and much less sugar. Even juice with pulp provides less fibre than whole fruit. Not only that, the fruit will help satisfy your hunger and the juice will not. If you pack a lunch for your kids or grandkids, try including a bottle of water and a piece of fruit instead of a juice box. Need some flavour for that water? Add some lemon or lime wedges.

Get cooking**

If you're like many busy modern women, you probably have the local pizza place on your speed dial. But delivery pizza—or even frozen pizza—is high in fat and sodium and often lacks fibre. You can make a healthier, portion-controlled version quickly and easily. I call it the Pita Pizza. Use a 6-inch whole-grain pita as your crust, add a low-sodium pizza sauce, lightly sprinkle on some low-fat mozzarella, and top it with your favourite veggies. Pop it in the oven or toaster until the cheese melts, and you're done—in way less time than it takes

---

**Quoted from the blog of Ashley Grachnik, RD, CDE, Registered Dietitian and Certified Diabetes Educator

for a delivery! And you can save even more time by buying pre-cut, washed veggies. You can control the portion by eating only one, and you can control the fat by limiting the amount of cheese and using more veggies.

This is just one example of how you can make healthier versions of your favourite take-out or restaurant choices at home. If you're looking for resources on healthy meal planning, you might consider cookbooks by Lucy Waverman, Bonnie Stern, and Rose Reisman.

Eat your fruits and veggies ... and your leafy greens

What's the dinnertime refrain you remember most vividly from childhood? For me it's my mother saying, "Eat your fruits and vegetables." She may not have known the science, but she definitely believed that fruits and vegetables promoted good health, and dessert often consisted of fresh fruit. As it turns out, we now know that vegetables contain essential nutrients we all need for optimal growth and health. We also know that people who eat more than two vegetable servings per day (versus one or none) are 40 percent more likely to experience a slower rate of age-related cognitive decline in late adulthood.

It's safe to say that all vegetables are good for you in this regard, but leafy greens such as collard greens, kale, rapini, spinach, and Swiss chard offer the most protection. And even if you're not a veggie lover, almost everyone has favourite fruits. One serving is not a lot of food: it's just a medium-sized apple or orange, for instance, a half-cup of cooked vegetables, or one cup of salad greens. Aim to consume at least seven servings of fruits and vegetables per day, the minimum recommended for adults in the Canada's Food Guide. Greens are great added to soups, pasta sauces, and chili. Top your pizza with arugula or kale. Get creative—you can do this!

Boost your vitamin B intake: Folate, B12, and B6

It would be hard to overemphasize the importance of getting enough of the B vitamins. Vitamin B12 and folate are needed to keep homocysteine from accumulating in the bloodstream. What is homocysteine and why does it matter? Unless you're a medical professional, you probably won't be familiar with this amino acid, but high levels of it in the blood can cause blockages in the arteries; that's why low levels of vitamin B12 and folate are associated with an increased risk of cognitive impairment and stroke. It is also important to get a balance of B vitamins, so be sure you also get B6. Food sources of the B vitamins include the following: for vitamin B12—meat, poultry, fish, dairy products, eggs, fortified soy, and fortified non-dairy milk; for folate—cooked spinach, lentils, black beans, broccoli, asparagus, artichokes, and avocados; and for vitamin B6— meat, poultry, fish, avocado, bananas, and baked potato.

I am conservative about the use of supplements; I firmly believe that in most circumstances they are no substitute for healthy food, but there are important exceptions. For instance,

I absolutely encourage pregnant women to take a multivitamin with adequate folate to protect from neurological disease in the growing fetus. And, as noted nutritionist and registered dietician Leslie Beck points out, multivitamins also provide minerals we may not get from our daily diets, such as selenium and zinc; therefore I recommend them for others as well.

I also recommend patients take vitamin D supplements every day. More on this in Chapter 7 in the discussion of osteoporosis.

Boost your vitamin E intake

Vitamin E is a powerful antioxidant that protects cells from oxidation and inflammation. It may also reduce breast cysts, an uncomfortable problem for women at various times of hormonal fluctuation, such as at adolescence and menopause. Best food sources for vitamin E are wheat germ oil, sunflower seeds, sunflower oil, safflower oil, grapeseed oil, hazelnuts, peanuts, and peanut butter.

Add polyphenol-rich foods

Have you ever heard of microglia? Again, unless you are a health professional your answer is probably a resounding *no!* Well, fair enough. Microglia are brain cells that remove toxic proteins that accumulate in the brain as we age. Polyphenols enhance the action of these cells, and they are also powerful antioxidants that can help protect brain cells from free radical damage. Good food sources of polyphenols include acai berries, blackberries, blueberries, cherries, cranberries, plums, pomegranate seeds, strawberries, raspberries, red grapes, and walnuts. Just one cup of berries or 14 walnut halves per day is enough to make a difference.

Increase your intake of omega-3 fatty acids

You have undoubtedly been aware of a lot of hype about omega-3 fatty acids. But it's not just hype. Higher intakes and higher blood levels of omega-3 fats are associated with reduced risk of coronary heart disease, stroke, and Alzheimer's. Twelve ounces per week of oily fish such as salmon, trout, char, and sardines provide the equivalent of about 1,000 milligrams per day—all you need. And here is another exception to my usual stance on supplements: if you don't eat fish, consider taking a fish oil supplement that contains at least 500 milligrams of omega-3s combined.

Reduce your fat intake

We need fat in our diets—in fact, we can't live well without it. Dietary fat is a necessary source of energy and of essential fatty acids our bodies can't make; it helps us absorb the fat-soluble vitamins A, D, E, and K, and it helps insulate our bodies and protect our hearts. However, there are good fats and bad fats. The bad ones are saturated fats that come from high-fat dairy products, butter, bacon fat, tropical oils, baked goods such as cookies and cakes, beef, processed meats with a high fat content—all of which are linked to increases in LDL cholesterol ("bad" cholesterol) blood levels, internal inflammation, and weight gain. For a person eating a 2,000-calorie-per-day diet, ingesting just 22 grams of saturated fat or less per day is associated with negative health outcomes. But there are sources of good fats, too, including avocados, whole eggs, nuts, fatty fish, chia seeds, and extra virgin olive oil.

Watch your cholesterol

As you undoubtedly know, there is "good cholesterol" and there is "bad cholesterol." Which is which and what is the difference? LDL, or low-density lipoprotein, is the bad cholesterol. It's the type that puts your heart at risk because it contributes to the build-up of plaque, a thick, hard deposit that can clog your arteries and cause atherosclerosis. So you want your LDL levels to be low. HDL, or high-density lipoprotein, is the good cholesterol, and higher levels of it are better. Experts believe HDL cholesterol may act in a variety of helpful ways that tend to reduce the risk for heart disease, including scavenging and removing LDL, and reducing, reusing, and recycling LDL by transporting it to the liver, where it can be reprocessed. (See Section A of the Appendix for guidelines on cholesterol levels.)

Get your daily calcium

Strong bones and strong teeth. That's what most people think when they hear the word *calcium*. And yes, about 99 percent of the calcium in our bodies is in our bones and teeth. It's the mineral that helps to build our bones and keep them healthy, just as it does for our teeth. But that is not the whole story by a long shot. Calcium also helps our blood clot, helps our nerves send and receive messages, and helps our muscles contract. Most people need 1,000 to 1,500 milligrams of calcium a day for optimal functioning of these systems. Decreasing levels of estrogen at menopause contribute to bone loss, so post-menopausal women need more calcium in order to maintain strength in the bone they have and help prevent osteoporosis.

Food sources of calcium include milk, yogurt (fat-free, please), and soy milk. Another good source of calcium is almonds: a handful (1/4 cup) contains about 80 milligrams of calcium and is also an excellent source of "healthy" fat. Vegetables such as broccoli and kale, and fish such as salmon, also provide calcium, but you would have to eat an awful lot to meet the daily requirements.

And here is the final exception to my conservative stance on supplements: if you're not able to have three servings of dairy per day, or if you're among the people who for any number of reasons find it hard to get the recommended 1,200 milligrams per day of calcium, I would suggest you take a calcium supplement to round up to 1,200 milligrams on the days on which your intake of dietary calcium falls significantly short. (And no, I don't work for the Dairy Farmers of Canada, but they are right: dairy products are a great, easy-to-absorb, dietary source of calcium.)

Whatever your source of calcium, be sure not to overdo it: too much calcium might increase the risk of kidney stones or interfere with the absorption of other vitamins and minerals. Be aware, too, that some recent research has linked excess calcium to calcification of the arteries to the heart, so more is not better.

Be cautious with caffeine

Millions of us rely on coffee to wake us up, keep us going, and improve concentration and focus. But how much is too much, and what is the difference between caffeine and coffee? Caffeine is a naturally occurring chemical found in more than 60 plants, including coffee beans, tea leaves, and kola nuts. It is also found in cacao pods, the source of chocolate products. Synthetic caffeine is sometimes added to foods, to soft drinks and energy drinks, and to medicines.

According to the Mayo Clinic, up to 400 milligrams of caffeine a day appears to be safe for most healthy adults— that's roughly the amount of caffeine in four cups of brewed coffee—but some people are more sensitive to caffeine than others. Too much caffeine can cause insomnia, headaches, irritability, and nervousness. If you're one of the sensitive ones, just small amounts of caffeine—even one cup of coffee or tea—may prompt unwanted effects such as restlessness, sleep problems, nervousness, and even heart palpitations. In fact, one of my patients rushed to a hospital emergency department with heart palpitations. When the doctor asked about her caffeine consumption, she said she drank a couple of cups of coffee every morning plus about 10 cans of diet cola every day. The diagnosis: heart palpitations due to excessive intake of caffeine. Case closed: when she reduced her caffeine consumption, the palpitations were remarkably reduced and she has felt much better ever since.

What about caffeine and kids? One hundred milligrams a day is the most a child should be allowed, but I certainly would not recommend that children be allowed to drink coffee.

Don't sneak that snack. Make it part of your eating plan!
That's right: make snacking an integral part of the way you eat. Just make sure your snacks are nutritious.

Snacking between meals can spell disaster for anyone who is trying to get down to or maintain a healthy weight. Why? Because most people snack on things that offer big rewards on the taste front but almost no rewards on the nutrition front—chips, candy bars, crackers. You get the picture. But including a healthy snack between meals is an excellent way to increase your nutritional intake and at the same time tame your appetite so that you're not ravenous at mealtime. So feel free to snack wisely, and by all means do not skip a meal. If your body is in starvation mode by the time you sit down to eat, you are much more likely to eat too quickly, which does not give your brain time to register the fact that you've eaten. The likely result is that you will overeat.

One effective snacking strategy is to have a big bowl of vegetable soup before you start preparing dinner; it keeps you from high-calorie, empty-calorie snacking while you cook. Or maybe purée the soup and drink a couple of cups—hot or cold—while you're cooking instead of drinking a glass or two of wine. It's basically just vegetables and water with a smattering of herbs (keep it low-salt or no-salt), and it will ensure that you're not ravenous when you sit down to eat.

Healthy snacks include such things as a dozen almonds and a piece of fruit, a half cup of yogurt with a cup of berries, an ounce and a half of low-fat cheese with two high-fibre crackers, and two high-fibre crackers with two tablespoons of natural peanut butter. These may not sound like much, but if you eat slowly and take time to enjoy them, these snacks will satisfy your between-meal hunger. And perhaps you've noticed that each one of them includes both protein and fibre—two essential elements of a healthy snack.

Order apps when eating out

Restaurant portions have gotten bigger and bigger over the years, to the point that many main courses are actually much more food than you need. Try ordering two appetizers instead of an entrée. Chances are your hunger will be satisfied. Alternatively, order an appetizer and share a main course. You can even share with yourself: just ask for a side plate, cut the portion served in half, and remove it from your plate. Then take it home and enjoy a wonderful supper the next night! If it's not on the plate in front of you, you'll be less likely to eat it from the second plate.

A Final Word on Healthy Eating and Diet

Our earth is bountiful, and so are our food factories, and it's up to each one of us to figure out the best way to take advantage of that bounty. Too much of a good thing is not good for us; overeating leads to overweight and obesity, with negative consequences for long-term health. The opposite is also true: too little of a good thing is not good for us; our societal emphasis on thinness, and all the ads that reinforce that emphasis, might make undereating seem like an attractive option. We need to be careful not to slip into disordered eating habits by eating either too much or too little. What we want to aim for is a kind of collaborative comfort with food, neither overindulging in comfort foods nor feeling uncomfortable about eating well to satisfy our normal, hearty appetites.

The motto of the recently revised and published Canada's Food Guide is "Eat Well. Live Well." Yes, that is what it is all about. Importantly, the guide focuses not only on *what* we eat but also on *how* we eat. We need to cook more often, be mindful, enjoy our food, and eat meals with others. By sharing meals and making them social occasions with good conversation, by avoiding fast food and not eating on the run, we will individually and as a nation do better and be healthier.

2

PUMP IT UP AND LET IT REST

Exercise and Sleep

I n Chapter 1 we talked about diet, one of the three most important factors we have control over when it comes to enhancing our health. Now let's talk about the other two: exercise and sleep.

Living Athletic: Making Exercise a Regular Part of Your Life

Just as some people hear the word *diet* and think, "Oh no! I don't want to starve myself," so too some hear the word *exercise* and think, "Oh no! Anything but the gym." But as you will remember, when we talk about diet we're talking about adopting a healthy, satisfying way of eating that we can sustain throughout our lives, not a quick weight-loss scheme that almost certainly will have only short-term results. Perhaps you won't be surprised, then, to learn that when we talk about exercise, at its most basic, we're simply talking about building regular activity into your life. And by regular I mean daily, if at all possible. It doesn't have to entail endless hours at the gym, running on the treadmill, pedalling through spinning classes, lifting weights, doing strenuous aerobics. All these things are good for us when they're done properly, but here's some good news: to maintain a basic level of fitness it is not absolutely necessary to do any of them.

So, at the start, one of most important things I want to say about exercise is that it definitely does *not* equal going to the gym. It means being active every day. It means adopting the "next subway stop" strategy—walking to the next stop rather than the one that's closest to your house. It means taking the stairs instead of the elevator, or if your office or condo is on a high floor, you might start by taking the stairs to the second floor and the elevator from there, and then work up to walking up two flights of stairs before you get on the elevator, and then three.

Exercise is going outside to play with your kids—or your grandkids. It's going to your local park, or going for a walk after dinner instead of driving to a movie—and if you really want to see that movie, how about walking around the block a couple of times before you get in the car?

I tell my patients that my definition of exercise involves thinking about activity in a positive way and making it a regular, voluntary part of their lives. I encourage them to think of being active as a way of living rather than as another item on their to-do list. After all, there is no 11th commandment: *Thou shalt exercise at least five out of every seven days.* Too often women think, "Okay, I have to go exercise now," and they do 20 minutes on the treadmill, while they're focused on a million other things they have to do, and so *having* to exercise is just one more stressor in their day. That is not what I mean by voluntary exercise. To be as beneficial as possible, exercise should help you decrease your stress level, not increase it. It should be something that helps you really enjoy your life.

Women often say to me, "Yes, Dr. Brown, I know. You've told me so many times that I need to exercise, but I just simply have no time." Saying "I have no time" is really saying "It's not my priority." Well, maybe today your kid is in the emergency department with a broken arm, so you're right, today exercise is not your priority. But if it's never your priority, all the research suggests that sooner or later you'll pay the price in compromised health.

One of my goals as a doctor who understands the benefits of exercise is to have women change their view of exercise and start to *live athletic*. But what does living athletic mean? It means working "athletic" into your self-image, thinking of athletic as the way you live, not as something you have to do. I'd love it if I never heard another patient tell me they simply have no time for exercise. I'd love it if instead they told me things that show they have made it a priority. Like the woman who told me she has started taking running shoes to work so she can go out for a good walk at lunchtime. And the woman who told me she now stays at work late one day and goes in early the next so that she doesn't feel guilty when she leaves a bit early that day to do a dance class. Why not try adjusting your work schedule in a similar way so that you can do a spinning class or a yoga class or whatever it is you like to do?

A lot of women these days lead hectic lives—getting the kids to school, fighting the subway crowds or the traffic at rush hour to get to work on time, fulfilling their responsibilities in often stressful work situations, picking up the kids from daycare and maybe carpooling them to sports practices or music lessons, making dinner, doing laundry, etc., etc., etc. Hectic, yes. But that kind of hectic activity is not the kind of activity that's going to enhance their health. It is regular, moderate aerobic exercise that pays rich dividends for long-term well-being.

But why exercise in the first place?

What exactly are those dividends? Fair question. So far I've been encouraging you to exercise because exercise is good for you, but I haven't told you precisely why it is good for you. So let's consider some of the major benefits of regular physical activity. Here is a short—and I hope persuasive—list of the benefits of living athletic. The science shows conclusively that physically active people

- live longer, healthier lives
- are more energetic
- are more productive
- are less likely to have chronic diseases such as type 2 diabetes, cancer, and heart disease
- are better able to cope with stress
- are more likely to enjoy prolonged independence as they age
- enjoy better balance and are less likely to fall
- report having better sex lives
- are less likely to have debilitating hot flashes

And that's not all. Some newer research links aerobic exercise with a decreased risk of dementia. Further, *New York Times* health columnist Aaron Carroll, who is a professor of paediatrics at Indiana University School of Medicine, wrote in June 2016 that exercise has been shown to have an amazingly positive impact on people with a large number of chronic diseases. He discusses multiple research studies that confirm many benefits of exercise, including the following:

- It reduces the pain and improves joint function in people with osteoarthritis of the knee.

- It increases aerobic capacity and muscle strength in patients with rheumatoid arthritis.
- It can lower blood pressure in people who have hypertension.
- It can lower cholesterol and triglyceride levels.
- It improves physical function of people with Parkinson's disease.
- It increases the distance that people with chronic obstructive pulmonary disease can walk and improves their overall ability to function.

The list goes on. Suffice it to say here that there is overwhelming evidence of many health benefits of exercise. We will talk in more depth about some of these benefits in the chapters that follow. We will look at some real-life examples of people for whom exercise has literally been a lifesaver. For now, though, let's figure out what level of exercise is right for you.

How much is enough?

The Heart and Stroke Foundation of Canada says that ideally we should all get 150 minutes per week of moderate exercise. That's just a baseline. The 150 minutes doesn't have to be 30 minutes in a row 5 days a week, although that is good for your heart.

You're not alone if you're saying to yourself, "Just what exactly is 'moderate' exercise?" There is a lot of confusion about how hard you have to exercise in order to enjoy substantial health benefits from it. There are all kinds of heart rate numbers we could look at, but the simple rule of thumb I usually tell people is this: you need to be a little sweaty and a little short of breath. If you're able to sing while you're walking your dog, you're not working hard enough. And don't forget, as the dog stops and starts, so does the dog walker, so she is not getting her heart rate up and keeping it up.

You don't see most people stopping and measuring their heart rate when they're exercising. Almost nobody does that, but anyone can tell—without having to measure—when they're a little bit sweaty and a little bit out of breath. If that describes you when you exercise, then you know you're working at a good heart rate for you. And by good I mean a heart rate that is going to be beneficial to your overall health.

So if you're not going to hit the gym, what can you do to live athletic? Start by setting your own goals and trying to achieve them. Your first goal may be just getting out the door. But a month later you may have a bigger, more ambitious goal than that, like getting out the door and walking around your block. And a month later maybe you'll walk around three times. Maybe you're one of the lucky women who live close to their workplace and you can walk 15 minutes to work and walk 15 minutes to get back home again. Or if you can't walk to work, this is a perfect time to put the "next subway stop" strategy into play. Perhaps you can map out a path in your neighbourhood and start walking it before or after dinner.

After about three or four weeks you should be able to do it faster, or better still, you should be able to go farther in the same amount of time.

Formal recommendations on how much and what type of exercise you should be getting, from the Canadian Society for Exercise Physiology and from the Heart and Stroke Foundation of Canada, can be found in Section B of the Appendix.

When it comes to exercise, embrace it and pace it

Don't be a weekend warrior. The research is unequivocal: being moderately active in your day-to-day life is beneficial to your health. You don't have to do high-intensity exercise. In fact, in some circumstances it can actually be counterproductive. Some women's schedules are so full and their lives so hectic (sound familiar?) that they adopt a "weekend warrior" exercise routine. Studies show that people who really push their level of exertion on the weekend to make up for the fact that they didn't have time to exercise during the week actually do themselves harm. At least one study has linked this type of exercise to an increased risk of heart attack. You can't make up on Saturday and Sunday what you didn't do Monday through Friday. The message about activity is simple: *embrace it and pace it.*

Making your health a priority

Ladies, let me close this discussion of exercise by asking you this: just how important to you is your own health?

You probably answered that question with an immediate, knee-jerk reaction, thinking to yourself that there is nothing more important. But when it comes to getting enough exercise, women often put themselves last on the priority list, even though they know the correlation between exercise and health. They tell themselves they'll get to it when they have done this and that, when they have taken care of their parents, when they are finished paying the bills, when they have done that little extra bit of work. And by putting themselves last on the list they are essentially saying, "My health is not my own priority." But think about this: when you're on a flight and the flight attendant is giving instructions about how to use the oxygen mask, what do they say? We've all heard this a thousand times, right? They always tell you that when the oxygen masks come down you should put one on yourself first and then put one on the child beside you because if you don't take care of yourself you won't be there to take care of your child.

The modern age is full of wonderful technology, and one of the bits of technology I find particularly useful in taking care of myself is the fitness tracker. Some may say I'm being obsessive, but I challenge myself to get in a certain number of steps each day. Before the fitness tracker, I assumed that I took enough steps in a busy day at the office, walking from room to room and barely sitting down. So when I started using it, I was astounded to find that a busy day at the office equals only about 4,000 steps—not nearly enough. So yes, when my workday is done, and after a break, I hop on the treadmill at home and keep moving until I reach my goal.

To Sleep, Perchance to Dream

I am not in the habit of quoting Shakespeare in my medical practice, but you have to admit he knew a thing or two about the restorative properties of sleep—even without the benefit of modern research. Just consider this quotation from Macbeth:

> *Sleep that knits up the ravell'd sleeve of care,*
> *The death of each day's life, sore labour's bath,*
> *Balm of hurt minds, great nature's second course,*
> *Chief nourisher in life's feast.*

In our hectic modern world we seem to have lost sight of how important sleep is. Not sleeping very much has come to be looked upon as a badge of honour. It's seen as an indication of how much you care about your work, how busy you are, how important you are, how productive you are. But we are beginning to understand that sleep deprivation is actually incredibly detrimental to your health … and eventually to your long-term productivity. Even in medicine there are now rules about how long interns can be awake when doing their shifts because they are dealing with life and death situations, and we know they cannot function properly without adequate sleep.

What sleep does ... and what not getting enough of it does

Although scientists have done extensive research to understand sleep and have discovered many important things about it, there is a great deal about how sleep works that remains very much a mystery. But there are some things we do know with certainty about this mysterious one-third of our lives: the research shows conclusively that adequate sleep is absolutely necessary to keeping us healthy and happy. For instance, we know that sleep is necessary for our nervous system to work properly. And we know that a sleeping body does not mean an inactive brain. Far from it. In fact, activity in the brain during sleep may exercise vital connections in the central nervous system and thus keep them from weakening.

We also know a thing or two about too little sleep. Too little sleep not only results in next-day sleepiness but also negatively affects concentration, memory, and the ability to perform physical tasks. When we don't get adequate sleep, our neurons begin to malfunction—they become polluted with by-products of normal cellular activity and, as a result, they become depleted of energy. Yet we continue to discount the importance of sleep.

Yes, not sleeping enough has become a societal norm, but I'm happy to say there seems to be an emerging societal backlash, a new focus on the importance of actually getting adequate sleep. This new focus on sleep really needs to address changes we can make to reverse unhealthy attitudes and behaviours, such as not caring about sleep, trying to prove we don't need very much sleep, going to bed too late, getting up too early, powering through our days at a less than optimal level of consciousness.

The sleep revolution

One powerful force in this backlash is Arianna Huffington, co-founder and editor-in-chief of *The Huffington Post*. Her book *The Sleep Revolution: Transforming Your Life, One Night at a Time* is based on an extensive review of current research on exactly what is going on when we sleep and dream. Ms. Huffington asserts that we are in the midst of a sleep deprivation crisis that is having profound consequences—on our health, our job performance, our relationships, and our happiness. And she knows about sleep deprivation first-hand.

She is the first to admit that she could have been a mascot for the "I don't need to sleep" crowd. A highly successful and driven journalist and businesswoman, she prided herself on how much she could get done in a day—a day that was made longer by the fact that her nights were so short. Then one day she woke up on her office floor, having passed out and fallen, in the process fracturing her face. That was her wake-up call. That is when she realized she had been riding the crest of a wave of exhaustion. And when the wave broke, so did she. Happily for the rest of us, she realized that hers was not a unique situation, and she set out to make the world aware of the dangers of too little sleep.

Doctors refer to strategies for improving sleep as sleep hygiene, and luckily for us, Ms. Huffington does more than decry the current state of sleeplessness in our society; she also offers strategies for getting more—and better—sleep. The ones I find most effective are these:

1. Create a bedroom environment that's dark, quiet, and cool.
2. Turn off electronic devices at least 30 minutes before bedtime.
3. Don't charge your phone next to your bed. Even better: Gently escort all devices completely out of your bedroom. And yes, you're better off if you avoid having a TV in the bedroom. It's much more likely to induce stress than to alleviate it as you become engrossed in suspenseful shows or provoked by the news of the day—neither of which will help you fall asleep.
4. Stop drinking caffeine after 2:00 p.m.
5. Use your bed for sleep and sex only—no work!
6. Take a hot bath with Epsom salts in the evening to help calm your mind and body.
7. Wear pyjamas, nightgowns, or even a special T-shirt—it'll send a sleep-friendly message to your body. If you wore it to the gym, don't wear it to bed.

8. Do some light stretching, deep breathing, yoga, or meditation to help your body and your mind transition to sleep.

9. Choose a real book or an e-reader that does not emit blue light if you like to read in bed. And make sure it's not work related: novels, poetry, philosophy— anything but work.

10. Sip chamomile or lavender tea to ease yourself into sleep mode.

Another standard element of sleep hygiene is establishing a regular sleep schedule. As with anything else, establishing a new health pattern takes time, so don't be discouraged if you find it hard to reset your sleep regime. Ideally you want to get on a schedule that gets you to bed at roughly the same time each night and out of bed at roughly the same time each morning. And yes (unfortunately perhaps), this includes weekends. Try to get up at the same time in the morning even if you have had a late night—consistency will help to regulate your circadian rhythms and make a good night's sleep more likely. Keep in mind that there are, of course, exceptions to every rule, but try to keep as regular a sleep schedule as possible.

Sleep problems

On the one hand are the people who decide not to sleep very much because they think it's a waste of time, and on the other are the people who long for a good night's sleep but just can't seem to get one. Even with proper sleep hygiene, some people still find it difficult to fall asleep or to stay asleep.

Too often their first approach to solving this problem is to take sleep medications. Depending on the individual situation, these medications can have their place in the medical treatment of sleep problems, but most medications that help you sleep have an addicting potential in the long run. Sleeping pills must be used with caution and, ideally for a very limited period of time.

It's usually helpful to look at sleep problems as a symptom and to try to discover the actual reason for them. Many sleep problems stem from an underlying cause that a person may not be aware of, and therefore a physician can often do more good by teasing out what is really going on than by simply writing a prescription.

The reason for disturbed sleep can be something as simple as the mom who is constantly listening for her kids in her sleep. If you were her when your children were small, then you may still be listening for every little noise, and therefore you somehow manage to stay in a light stage of sleep and don't get the kind of deep, restorative sleep we all need. Well, you may just need to be reminded that your kids are grown now and out of the house, so there is really no need to be listening for them anymore. Sure, it is a habit that you developed over years, and even though habits can be hard to break, once you're aware of it you can break it.

Perhaps it is an issue of anxiety that's not letting you sleep. Maybe it's an issue of hormonal imbalance, so you're waking up sweating 10 times a night. Or it may be situational—someone just died in your family and you don't seem able to cope. Once we uncover the problem, the right strategy usually becomes evident and resolution soon follows. Occasionally, however, we can't find the problem, and so we send someone to a sleep clinic, to a sleep specialist, to a sleep respirologist, or to a psychiatrist who has expertise in sleep disorders to help them find out why they're not sleeping—or if they are sleeping, to find out why they're waking up tired.

Often the answer is sleep apnea, a potentially serious condition in which a person's breathing stops and restarts repeatedly throughout the night. These pauses in breathing can last anywhere from a second or two to several minutes, and when normal breathing starts again it often starts with a loud snort or choking sound. Sleep apnea can be very serious: it can lead to high blood pressure and heart problems, type 2 diabetes, metabolic syndrome, and complications with medications and surgery.

You should be aware that sleep is not just about you but also about who you're sleeping with. Heavy snoring can be an indicator of sleep apnea, so if your partner is a snorer who keeps you awake at night, it is not okay to say, "Okay, I'll just put in earplugs and his snoring won't bother me." If your partner's sleeping is disturbed—and therefore disturbing you—it's not just for you that he should be assessed; it's also for his own health.

Anxiety sabotages sleep, as I suggested above, but it's not always easy to find the cause of the anxiety. One patient in her late 60s had never slept well, even as a child. Joannie always had trouble falling asleep and she always had trouble staying asleep. She said, "In the daytime I'm always tired, but when night falls I'm totally wired." I won't say it was easy to discover the underlying problem—obviously it was not easy or it would not have taken her until she was in her 60s to do so. But with the help of a therapist she finally did discover it. When she was just 3½ years old, her mother contracted tuberculosis and had to spend 18 months in a sanatorium, so Joannie was sent to live with relatives. Her chief caregiver was a strict and unforgiving woman, and if Joannie refused to go to sleep at bedtime, the caregiver put a pillow over her head until she passed out. This happened repeatedly throughout the time she was away from her own home.

No wonder she had trouble sleeping! Joannie's therapist suggested a strategy to counteract Joannie's anxiety about sleep. She suggested that each night at bedtime, before turning out the light and getting into bed, Joannie should look around her room and say to herself, "This is my own bedroom in my own home. This is a safe place. I am safe here. No one is going to come in and put a pillow over my head. I do not need to be on guard. I want to sleep now, and I can sleep safely here." Joannie says that this strategy worked the very first night she tried it and it has worked every night since. And she muses about how different her life might have been if only she had met that therapist when she was younger.

Staying Active and Resting Well

We've now reviewed the importance of healthy eating, exercise, and being more active, as well as the importance of sleeping well and feeling rested and refreshed in the morning. Sounds so simple. But, in truth, any change is difficult at first. We often deliberate about making healthy lifestyle choices for a long time before we begin to adopt them. Sometimes we adopt them only once our health has failed and the changes are more or less forced on us. But wouldn't it be better to embrace these healthy choices *before* anything goes wrong … so that we're doing everything in our power to ensure nothing does go wrong? Of course it would.

Perhaps not quite as simple as it sounds, but living a healthy lifestyle is an achievable goal. And once achieved it can become almost second nature to remain focused and maintain healthy habits without having to exert enormous ongoing effort. Others have done it, and you can, too!

3

HEALTHY HEMISPHERES

The Aging Brain

You may wonder why, after covering diet, exercise, and sleep in the introductory chapters of a book on women's health, I chose to place the chapter on brain health as the first of the chapters on specific organs and bodily systems. My first reason is a simple one. The brain is the alpha and the omega of life: without brain function there can be no life outside the womb, and the cessation of brain function is the medically accepted definition of death.

My second reason is to answer a question I hear repeatedly: But aren't women's and men's brains the same? Many people think they are, and until quite recently there was little scientific evidence to the contrary. That idea is rapidly changing. We are very far behind in brain research compared to research on many other organ systems. In fact, we are probably now about where we were in our understanding of the cardiovascular system some 30 years ago. One thing is for certain, though: we're beginning to appreciate that there are, in fact, gender differences in brain structure, brain function, and brain health.

What's the Difference?

It is true that the topic of gender differences between men's and women's brains is controversial and that not all researchers find the same results. If you're skeptical about such differences, though, just consider this paragraph from an article from Columbia University on how gender differences in brain structure may affect human function:

> Women tend to be better at sensing emotional messages in conversations, gestures, and facial expressions, and are thus more sensitive. Women start to speak and read at an earlier age than men and are generally better in verbal skills, such as learning a different language. They tend to have a better grasp on grammar and spelling, and girls have better handwriting than boys do. Women have better sight at night and have a more acute sense of smell, taste, and hearing. Men are better at spatial coordination and have a better sense of direction (usually!). They excel in math and are great at

interpreting three-dimensional objects. They have better hand-eye coordination and more precise control of large muscle movement. They have poor peripheral vision but better sight in bright light and better sense of perspective.... These differences are not rules.... [But w]hen looking at large populations, these differences between men and women become evident, and proper statistical analysis takes care of the exceptions.

We are learning, for instance, that different parts of the brain light up differently in women than they do in men, given the same stimulus. With vision, for example, as suggested above, we know that men tend to see straight ahead farther and with greater perspective than women, while women tend to have better peripheral vision than men. This difference may go back to the time of hunters and gatherers when men were hunting for food and needed to spot their prey, and women needed to see what was happening all around them to protect their young. As your mother may have said, "I know what you're up to. I have eyes in the back of my head."

Men also have a greater sensitivity to fast-moving objects while women have better colour vision. And for the record: a man's resting brain is only 30 percent active while a woman's resting brain is 90 percent active. In other words, our brains are more active than men's even when we're resting. When men speak, only one brain area is activated, but when women speak our hearing areas are also activated; that's right—we can listen even while we're talking!

So, yes, we are learning that there are substantial differences both anatomically and physiologically between men's brains and women's brains, and therefore differences between men and women in brain health. What is the difference between physiological and anatomical? It's the classic structure-versus-function distinction. When I say physiological, I'm referring to how the brain functions, and when I say anatomical I'm referring to the structure of the brain—that is, how much grey matter and how much white matter there is, the relative sizes of brain structures, and differences in the density of neurons in particular structures. The proportions of grey and white matter are different in men and women. This does not imply a difference in intelligence, but it may play a part in the fact that women process information in a slightly different way than men do, even if they reach the same conclusions in the end.

It is only by studying these and other gender differences in the brain that we will get a better handle on why women are doing worse than men with regard to brain diseases, why 16 percent of women age 71 and older have Alzheimer's or other dementias compared to just 11 percent of men, why 70 percent of new Alzheimer's cases will be women, why women suffer more from depression and from diseases like MS and other neurological diseases.

Here is one dramatic example of things we have learned that have a direct bearing on women's brain health. As the excerpt from the Columbia article mentions, women have much better verbal memory and verbal skills than men do. This may be an advantage in many circumstances, but when we're looking for signs of early cognitive decline it is a disadvantage. Why? Dr. Pauline Maki and her group at the University of Illinois at Chicago may have the answer. They have done some fascinating research on clinical memory tests that measure an individual's ability to learn and remember a list of spoken words. These tests are widely used to diagnose dementia. What they found is that because of their above-mentioned advantage in verbal skills, women generally show better memory for this verbal material than men. In clinical practice, however, this gender difference is not taken into account. A woman who scores in the low normal range overall is actually scoring in the impaired range for women. Conversely, a man who scores in the impaired range overall could actually be in the low normal range for men.

This is problematic because in these settings the woman is often told she is fine and the man is told he is impaired, when in reality she is impaired and he is fine. Dr. Maki estimates that these errors occur 20 percent of the time. Therefore, given the common verbal memory advantage that women possess, Dr. Maki suggests that testing should be scored differently for men and women. Indeed, the present testing protocol disadvantages women since the drugs that are currently used for dementia tend to have the best impact early in the disease. Cognitive changes for women would be recognized earlier if the testing and scoring were more gender specific. It is also a disadvantage to men who are told that they are impaired when they are not. Women and men are simply not the same, and we need to be vigilant to ensure that no one is being disadvantaged by these gender differences.

Women's Brain Health Initiative

But that isn't the whole story. Thanks in large part to the work of Women's Brain Health Initiative (WBHI), science is now paying a lot of attention to women's brain health. WBHI is a partner of the Canadian Consortium on Neurodegeneration and Aging, which is an umbrella group that oversees all the brain research happening in Canada. Because of its significant funding clout, WBHI has been able to ensure that every participant group—in all brain research undertaken in Canada—includes enough women to matter. What do I mean by "enough women to matter"? I mean that there have to be enough women in each study to be statistically significant so the research conclusions of the study apply to women, not just to men.

And it isn't that women are a priority only in the research being done today. Governments come and go and researchers' interests shift, and those changes can also alter research priorities. But WBHI has been able to make sex and gender—and therefore women—part of the core value of all the brain research going on. And core values are impervious to the fickle winds of change. We may not know today why more women than men suffer from Alzheimer's, but because of the inclusion of women as a core value in research we *will know* at some point in the future.

In fact, there's a lot of research going on now to discover ways to identify cognitive decline earlier in women. This includes research on issues concerning Alzheimer's disease, which is now being recognized as "a woman's disease" because so many more women than men suffer from it, as mentioned above. Drug development is another important area of research because the drugs we currently have for treating brain problems may not work as effectively in women as they do in men.

The current research also includes a focus on lifestyle choices. We know some of the things that can contribute to cognitive difficulties in old age, and many of them are things we can control. For instance, we know we can alter smoking, diet, exercise, stress, blood pressure, and blood sugar levels—all of which can have a big impact on cognitive health, or to put it another way, on cognitive decline. As with any research, there is always the possibility of unexpected results. For instance, one study showed that the most important decade of life to affect brain health through exercise is your 20s. That's right, exercise in your 20s makes the biggest difference to your brain 50 years later! So, realistically, you are never too young to start thinking about your brain and how to keep it healthy.

Two Hemispheres, Two Hormones, One Brain

It is beyond the scope of this book to discuss all the hormones that have an impact on the brain, but there are two that you absolutely should be aware of: cortisol and estrogen.

Cortisol: The mess of stress

Stress can be a good thing or a bad thing. At a certain level it can be a benign motivator, giving us the focus and the energy to accomplish important tasks. In extraordinary circumstances, even a high level of stress can be beneficial: for instance, it can help the brain cope with life-threatening situations. But too much stress, and especially too much stress over a prolonged period of time, is harmful.

The human brain is wonderfully plastic: it actually changes with events, forming new neural pathways and deleting others, depending on an individual's experiences. But sustained, longer-term stress raises the level of the stress hormone *cortisol* in the blood, and excessive cortisol compromises the brain's ability to adapt. For example, among other things, it affects brain cells in the hippocampus, the area of the brain responsible for episodic memory. This and other stress-related changes in the brain make you more vulnerable to and less able to recover from insults to the brain such as strokes. Compared to younger individuals, older subjects in general show a larger cortisol response to challenge, but the effect of age on cortisol response is almost three-fold stronger in women than in men. This places women at greater risk of developing some age-related and stress-affected diseases, such as Alzheimer's and other dementias.

Estrogen: Good for your brain

Some research shows that the female hormone estrogen can be neuroprotective. In other words, it helps to salvage, recover, or aid in the regeneration of the nervous system, its cells, structures, and functions. We know that women who undergo estrogen hormone therapy early in menopause are less likely to develop cognitive impairment, including Alzheimer's and other dementias.

I discuss menopause, healthy aging, and hormone therapy in Chapter 5. However, if you are wondering whether hormone therapy is safe, the answer is a qualified yes. Initiating hormone therapy is now considered an acceptable option for relatively young women (up to age 59) and for healthy women who are bothered by menopausal symptoms if they are within ten years of menopause. There is increasing evidence that estrogen treatment/hormone therapy initiated during the premenopausal/early postmenopausal stage may inhibit the progression of atherosclerosis. Atherosclerosis is a disease in which plaque builds up inside your arteries. Your brain needs a constant flow of oxygen-rich blood and other nutrients, and clogged arteries slow down the flow of blood—to your heart, your brain, and other parts of your body. So hormone therapy has the potential to be useful in the prevention of early dementia and Alzheimer's; we know, for example, that women who undergo removal of their ovaries at a young age, perhaps to prevent a cancer, are more at risk for heart disease and Alzheimer's than the general population, unless they receive hormone therapy.

And estrogen also acts to relieve hot flashes and night sweats! More on that to follow.

Health Strategies for an Aging Brain

There are no guarantees a healthy lifestyle will absolutely prevent Alzheimer's or other dementias. But healthy lifestyle choices absolutely will improve blood flow to the brain, and that is a key component of maintaining a healthy brain. By making wise lifestyle choices today you can improve your chances of sustaining long-term brain health in later years. Here are five essential strategies.

1. Exercise

Exercise is an important component of all aspects of healthy aging. Brain health is no exception. You will remember from Chapter 2 that you don't have to become a "gym rat" in order to do the kind of exercise that confers solid health benefits. Moderate, sustained aerobic activity, ideally on a daily basis, is all it takes. For most of us, though, seven days a week is a big commitment and may not be practical or achievable. However, you can set a reasonable weekly goal: the objective here is to get more blood circulating through the brain regularly.

Thirty minutes a day of sustained aerobic exercise such as running will increase brain health, neural plasticity, brain function, and cognition. This kind of exercise is associated with the growth and creation of new brain cells, and that helps increase the volume of your brain.

The research also shows that exercise increases the level of brain-derived neurotropic factor (BDNF). Easy for me to say, right? BDNF is a protein that acts on the neurons of the central and peripheral nervous systems. It helps to support the survival of existing neurons and encourages the growth and differentiation of new neurons and synapses—functions that are critical to learning, memory, and neural plasticity (the brain's ability to continue to change and adapt).

As we age, our brain function and cognition are essential to maintaining an independent and healthy life. So I'll say it again: Exercise helps! For example, take a look at the effect exercise has on blood flow to the hippocampus (see Figure 1). This exciting picture illustrates the effect of exercise on blood flow to that region. The top photo (a) shows blood flow after exercise, and the bottom photo (b) shows blood flow before exercise. It is easy to see that exercise has greatly increased the amount of blood flow. Increased blood flow brings nutrients and oxygen to the brain and results in better brain function overall.

There is also evidence from a New York study by G. Ravaglia and colleagues, published in the journal *Neurology*

Figure 1: The Effect Exercise Has on Blood Flow to the
Hippocampus

a)

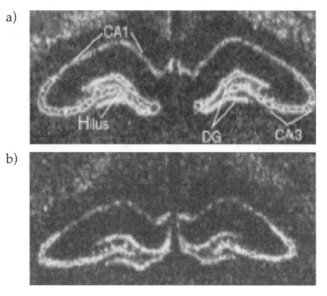

b)

Source: From CW Cotman, et al. Exercice: A Behavioural Intervention to
Enhance Brain Health and Plasticity. Trends in Neurosciences. 25(6):295-301,
2002. Used by permission.

(December 2007), that those who work out regularly are less
likely to get Alzheimer's. And a recent European study has
proven that there is a positive correlation between increased
exercise and reduction in stroke risk.

Patients sometimes ask me about the benefits of weight
training and interval training. Both of these are good for other
parts of your body, such as your muscles and your heart, but
there is no indication that they have the kind of positive effect
on your brain that aerobic exercise does.

2. Meditation and brain power

The practice of mindfulness meditation has moved: once found only in yoga studios and on the new-age fringes, it has now taken a place in mainstream medicine. Mindfulness applications are now routinely used to reduce and manage stress, depression, chronic pain, and other chronic health conditions.

In mindfulness training, individuals learn to focus their attention on what is happening in the present moment. They usually start by paying attention to their breathing, by simply becoming aware of each in-breath and each out-breath. Mindfulness allows for a nonjudgmental awareness of sensations, feelings, and states of mind—it lets people be aware of their thoughts but not get carried away by them.

Scientists have known for some time that meditation is a very effective technique for alleviating conditions like anxiety and depression, both of which, if left unchecked, are risk factors that increase the susceptibility to Alzheimer's and other dementias. Only relatively recently, though, have they discovered that meditation directly affects our grey matter.

Yes, it actually changes the human brain: people who meditate experience changes in brain structure that those who do not meditate do not experience. The evidence suggests that mindfulness meditation can also increase the structural connectivity between brain areas, as measured by white matter tracts in the brain, and that it can decrease the rate of cellular aging.

And now a landmark study has shown not only that meditation can change our brains for the better but also that it can do so in just eight weeks—even if we have never meditated before. It seems it is never too late or too onerous to learn brain-healthy practices.

The website food.ndtv.com describes this study as follows. In a study published in *Psychiatry Research: Neuroimaging*, U.S. researchers measured the brains of 16 people who had never meditated before and then again after they had completed an eight-week meditation program. During that time, the group spent an average of 27 minutes a day practising mindfulness meditation. At the end of the study the researchers found there was increased grey-matter density in the hippocampus, an area of the brain associated with learning and memory, and in other brain structures associated with self-awareness, compassion, and introspection. There was also a reduction in the size of the amygdala, the part of the brain that registers anxiety and stress.

In addition, a UCLA study published in 2009 that used high-resolution magnetic resonance imaging (MRI) to scan participants' brains found increased volumes in the brain regions known for regulating emotions—the hippocampus and areas within the orbitofrontal cortex, the thalamus, and the inferior temporal gyrus—in long-term meditators (who used various meditation techniques) compared to non-meditators. The implication is clear: meditation can lead to a calmer existence due to enhanced emotional control that is tied directly to changes in the brain that are caused by the meditation itself. No wonder meditation is prescribed as a stress reliever!

Meditation is an area of medical treatment that is rapidly evolving as we learn more about its benefits. To test it for yourself, you might want to try this five-minute mindfulness meditation practice, recommended at **www.bodyand soul.com**:

- Sit on the floor or on a chair. Make sure your back is straight and arms relaxed. Or, if it is more comfortable for you, lie on the floor.
- Bring your attention to your breath for one minute. Feel how your belly rises and falls.
- Widen your attention to include all your bodily sensations and any thoughts or feelings you may be having.
- Try to be a neutral observer of your thoughts and feelings. If you find yourself swept up in a train of thought or emotion, just return to focusing on your breath.

(For more about the benefits of meditation, I also recommend the following website: **www.mindful.org/meditation/ mindfulness-getting-started/**.)

Bottom line: reducing your levels of stress through activities like exercise and meditation can decrease the rate of cellular aging and therefore decrease your risk of developing Alzheimer's and other dementia.

3. Diet (again): Eat well for your brain to age well

Your brain is one of the most active parts of your body. Although it comprises only about 2 percent of your total body weight, it receives about 15 to 20 percent of your body's blood supply, and as you know, it is your blood that supplies the oxygen and the nutrients your body and brain need to function properly.

Remember the old saying "You are what you eat"? Well, it turns out it's true. Whatever you ingest nourishes—or fails to nourish—your brain and all other parts of your body. So let's take a look at how what we eat affects brain health.

I mentioned in Chapter 1 that the dinnertime refrain I remember most from my childhood is my mother saying, "Eat your fruits and vegetables." What I did not mention there is that my mother was also very clever in getting us to be interested in vegetables. When we were very young children, and long before it was fashionable, she made some meals as a "vegetable plate." She made a game out of how many vibrantly coloured veggies she could place on the plate ... and then she engaged us in the game of naming and spelling the names of all the vegetables! She knew we loved fruit, so she didn't need to devise a strategy to make fruits interesting.

Although our vegetable plates were a fun source of cognitive challenge and gain, I'm sure my mother did not know the science that shows a diet rich in vegetables reduces the risk of cognitive problems when compared to a diet that includes fewer vegetables. And the rate of cognitive decline is the lowest in women who eat the most cruciferous vegetables, such as broccoli, cauliflower, Brussels sprouts, cabbage, bok choy, and dark leafy greens. Research also makes clear that there is a positive correlation between BMI and the rate of cognitive decline: the greater the weight, the faster the decline—so you could say there is a neurological reason to control your weight through healthy diet and exercise.

Luckily for all of us women, scientific interest in nutrition and brain health has led to development of several diets designed for overall health, including brain health. Two of them emerge as the best dietary strategies for slowing down your brain's rate of aging and avoiding potential cognitive decline: the Mediterranean Diet and the MIND Diet. (For a detailed description of the MIND diet, and for links to more information about the Mediterranean and DASH diets, please see Section A in the Appendix.)

The Mediterranean diet

The Mediterranean diet was developed to mimic the diet of people who live in countries on the Mediterranean Sea because those populations were found to enjoy excellent heart health. It emphasizes fresh fruits and vegetables, low-fat or non-fat dairy products, fish, and whole grains. It not only allows but also actually recommends that wine be consumed in low to moderate amounts. Olive oil is the primary source of fat, and the recommended range of total daily fat intake is between 25 and 35 percent of total calories, with saturated fat no more than 7 percent of calories.

If it was developed for heart health, does it also work for brain health? Let's look at the science to answer that question. Researchers from Columbia University Medical Center asked nearly 700 people, most of whom were around age 80, to fill out a questionnaire about what they ate over the past year. They then divided the men and women into two groups: one that closely followed the Mediterranean diet and one that followed just a few of the diet's components. They did brain scans to measure the brain volume of each of the participants, and after about seven months they did brain scans again. The results? Those in the group who followed the Mediterranean diet more closely had less brain atrophy, which made their brains appear to be five years younger than the brains of people in the other group.

Researchers believe the beneficial effects of the Mediterranean diet on cognition likely stem from the abundance of foods rich in antioxidants (such as blueberries) and the anti-inflammatory action of foods such as whole grains, nuts, and vegetables. The fact that there is very little fatty red meat in this diet is also believed to be a factor.

The MIND diet

The MIND diet is a hybrid of the Mediterranean diet and the DASH diet. DASH is an acronym for Dietary Approaches to Stop Hypertension. As implied by the name, DASH was originally developed as a non-medical intervention to treat hypertension; it is based on research sponsored by the U.S. National Institutes of Health. Research shows that both the Mediterranean and the DASH diets reduce the risk of hypertension, heart attack, and stroke and also provide some protection against dementia.

MIND, of course, is also acronym; it stands for Mediterranean-DASH Intervention for Neurodegenerative Delay. It is based on years' worth of research about the foods and nutrients that have good—and bad—effects on the functioning of the brain over time. This relatively new diet could significantly lower a person's risk of developing Alzheimer's disease, even if it is not meticulously followed. So say the developers of the diet—nutritional epidemiologist Martha Clare Morris and her colleagues at Rush University Medical Center in Chicago—in a paper published in the online journal *Alzheimer's & Dementia: The Journal of the Alzheimer's Association*.

Their study showed that the MIND diet lowered the risk of Alzheimer's by as much as 53 percent in participants who adhered to the diet rigorously and by about 35 percent in those who followed it moderately well. The researchers got interesting results when they compared the MIND with the Mediterranean and the DASH diets. These diets were also found to reduce the incidence of Alzheimer's when followed meticulously—54 percent and 39 percent, respectively—but the benefit from moderate adherence to either of them was negligible.

Yes, it takes meticulous adherence to get the greatest benefit, but the good news is that the MIND diet is easier to follow. It includes 10 "brain-healthy food groups": green leafy vegetables, other vegetables, nuts, berries, beans, whole grains, fish, poultry, olive oil, and wine, and it cautions against five unhealthy food groups: red meats, butter and stick margarine, cheese, pastries and sweets, and fried or fast foods. It is interesting to note that berries are the only fruit specifically to be recommended in the MIND diet. "Blueberries are one of the more potent foods in terms of protecting of the brain," according to Dr. Morris. Strawberries have also performed well in past studies of the effect of food on cognitive function.

4. Smoking

We've talked about three things you can do to increase blood flow to the brain, decrease your stressors, and promote long-term brain health: exercise, meditate, and make wise eating choices. Now let's look at something you should avoid if you are serious about maintaining optimal brain function as you age: smoking.

You will probably not be surprised to hear me say that when it comes to smoking there is really very little to discuss. It is an absolute no! Smoking alters the diameter of blood vessels, causing constriction that limits the flow of blood—and therefore of oxygen—to the brain. There is an abundance of research that confirms the horrific harm that smoking causes. It damages memory, learning, and reasoning. And there is no safe amount: even one or two cigarettes a day will double your risk of heart disease. Quitting is difficult, some say more difficult than kicking a heroin habit. But it can be done! And it must be done! A number of over-the-counter patches, gums, nasal sprays, and prescription drugs are designed to help people quit smoking. Some people have had success with hypnosis. I cannot encourage you strongly enough to do whatever it takes for you to be tobacco free. And the sooner the better!

5. Alcohol

Excessive long-term alcohol consumption can result in neuro-logic damage and impaired mental processing, so obviously it is another thing to avoid. The medical advice is unanimous: limit your drinking. Notice I say limit your drinking, not stop drinking. Why? Because the research shows that moderate drinking can have beneficial health effects. For instance, there is a lot of research about the protective effects of red wine due to the presence in it of resveratrol, an antioxidant that helps reduce the amount of plaque build-up in your arteries. Generally, women are advised to limit alcohol consumption to one serving a day. Occasionally two. And remember: a serving is five ounces, not eight.

It's widely recognized in North America that we simply do not get enough sleep. Sleep problems affect as much as half the total adult population, and in older adults insufficient sleep is associated with increased risk of dementia. Yet many people don't realize that alcohol can have a seriously disruptive effect on a person's ability to get a good night's sleep.

Women's Brain Health Initiative cites a study published in the journal *Neurology*, in which MRI scans were used to determine whether sleep problems were linked to declining brain volume in a sample of 147 community-dwelling adults aged between 20 and 84. Poor sleep quality was associated with an increased rate of decline in the brain. The consensus is that we need about seven hours of uninterrupted sleep each night. Research shows that people who get fewer than seven hours of sleep have difficulty concentrating, and shorter hours of sleep may speed up the brain-aging process. So if you drink and you have trouble sleeping, the alcohol may be a contributing factor. I'm not an abolitionist by any means, but try a couple of weeks without alcohol and see if your sleep improves.

The Montreal Cognitive Assessment: The MoCA Test

So far in this chapter we have looked at important lifestyle issues and healthy strategies to promote brain health as we age and to delay aging-related deterioration of the brain. But if you're a younger woman who is concerned about your brain health right now, there is something you can do immediately to determine whether your concerns are warranted.

What are your first steps? Well, as you know, I'm a family doctor, and therefore I'm totally biased in that I believe Step 1 is to visit your family doctor. Get your blood pressure checked; have blood tests done for various diseases (have your thyroid function checked, as it can affect brain health); and ask for a full examination to evaluate any other potential risk areas that can be modified, such as your blood sugar levels, cholesterol, and weight/BMI. As part of an office assessment to review your physical health, your doctor can also do a cognitive assessment to evaluate your brain health.

In fact, there is a simple, 20-minute evaluation that can be done in the doctor's office—the MoCA Test is a 1-page, 30-point test that was developed in Montreal in 1996; it is used to test for significant memory loss and early Alzheimer's disease.

A poor score on the test may mean you require further assessment and perhaps intervention. Be aware, though, that anxiety, depression, changes in eyesight and/or hearing, and certain medications can also affect your performance. Let me say again, the best strategy is to have a talk with your doctor. If you are diagnosed with early cognitive decline, the medical aim will be to slow down the process as any loss that has already occurred cannot be reversed. We do know today that a combination of lifestyle intervention, medication, and support can help.

It Is Never Too Late to Start

A final word. The bottom line, ladies, is that our grey matter matters. We need to make our own health a priority and make lifestyle adjustments that ensure we are functioning at our very best, right now. And we need to make those important decisions to protect ourselves for the future so that we can enjoy full function, independence, and joyful living as we age.

Clearly, the younger you are when you choose healthy options, the better protection you will have in the long run, but it is never too late for healthy changes to result in a meaningful degree of benefit.

Yes, some of us are fighting an unfortunate genetic profile or harmful environmental exposures (such as second-hand smoke when we were kids) and other issues that are out of our control. But we really need to make the very best choices when it comes to the major modifiable factors that affect our long-term health. Will we be good, better, or best as we age? The answer is that a lot of it is up to us!

4

THE VALUE
OF VACCINES

Immunization-
Preventable Diseases

I f you're like most people, you think of your doctor as someone you need to see when you're sick, but a physician's job involves much more than curing illness. In fact, one of the most exciting things I do as a family doctor is to prevent disease. A big part of that prevention is educating patients about their health, giving them the information they need to make healthy lifestyle choices. But perhaps the most concrete, clear-cut way I keep my patients healthy is by immunizing them against vaccine-preventable diseases.

It's Wise to Immunize

Sometimes it's a little bit uncomfortable … but not for very long. For instance, when I immunize an infant for measles, mumps, and rubella, my office fills with that baby's wailing, and tears run down those chubby cheeks. And yet, despite knowing I have caused the child's momentary discomfort, I feel fantastic because I know that what I've just done may save that child's life.

I remember, albeit many years ago, doing rounds as a medical student at the Montreal Children's Hospital with the pediatrician on call. We walked into one room and found a child on a respirator, doing very poorly. She had diphtheria, a disease that affects a membrane on your trachea and blocks your breathing. I have never forgotten the wisdom in the doctor's words as he said, "Better the baby cries for five minutes after a shot than the parents cry for a lifetime." It is a very special message that I share with parents almost every day.

You only have to see one or two deaths from a vaccine-preventable disease to really appreciate what you are doing as a physician when you vaccinate a patient. In the course of my many years as a physician, I've been peripherally involved in a death by meningitis, and I've seen deaths from cervical cancer, deaths from anal cancers, deaths from pneumonia. I've seen cases of oral cancers and horrendous outcomes from the shingles disease. And all of these could have been prevented by effective, timely immunization. We lose adults to influenza every single year, in every province, every city, every hospital, even with good care and various medications; so many of those deaths could be prevented with the flu vaccine.

That undoubtedly helps to explain why I feel entirely grat-
ified and empowered as a physician when I talk to patients
about vaccine-preventable disease. When I vaccinate them I
know that as they are walking out my door I have given them
something that's really protective, really important to their
long-term health. I've given them the armour they need to fend
off a potentially fatal joust with menacing microbes: I've given
them a javelin they can rely on. I know that they're significantly
less likely to die of a vaccine-preventable disease than someone
who is not vaccinated. I often say to myself, "Not on my watch.
It's just not going to happen to one of my patients."

Vaccines are wonderful, but there are limitations to their
effectiveness when they're given to adults. Because of children's strong immune systems, we can generally eradicate
a disease with proper immunization. Think about polio, for
example. If your child has been immunized, he or she will
not get the disease. The same is true for you if you were
immunized when you were young. The vaccine is wonderfully effective in children, almost miraculously so. In adults,
however, immunization generally does not eradicate or eliminate the disease entirely. Rather, it attenuates the severity of
the disease, essentially making it less harmful, and cases of
polio in an immunized individual are very rarely lethal. So
whether we're talking about influenza or pneumonia or shingles, immunization does not prevent every episode of illness,
but if you become ill you will not become as sick as you would
if you had not been immunized. So yes, you may still get the

flu after a flu shot, but chances are really good that you will not end up in the emergency room, be admitted to the ICU, and die on a ventilator as the influenza virus overwhelms your immune system.

So if you walk out of your doctor's office after getting a vaccine and think to yourself, "Whew, I'm never going to get this disease!" but then you do get a mild case, please realize this is not a vaccine failure. It's not an unexpected occurrence because as we age our immune response is simply not as robust as a child's. When a patient comes to me and complains that they got the flu shot and then got the flu anyway, I say to them, "Yes, you got the flu, but you're here to tell me about it! That's what the vaccine accomplished!"

When you as a parent decided to have your child immunized, you opted to give them the most powerful protection we have against disease. Good for you! But many women seem to stop thinking about vaccination once their children have completed all their immunizations. That is a mistake; vaccines are not just for kids. There are vaccines that *you* need, vaccines that will continue to protect your health as you age. What are they? We'll get to that soon, but first let's look at the immune system and how vaccines work.

The question of how vaccines work is top of mind around the world as people everywhere deal with a new coronavirus, COVID-19, and follow the urgent global effort to create a vaccine that protects against it. We have been extremely successful since the 1950s in creating safe and effective vaccines against a number of viruses that cause potentially serious illnesses, including measles, mumps, rubella, and varicella (chicken pox).

Our immune system is always turned on, watching for invaders that pose a risk to our health—COVID-19 is a timely example. And vaccines help boost our own immune response.

The immune system's first line of defence against pathogens is the skin, which is highly resistant to viruses and bacteria. But many viruses can invade the body through the mucous membranes of the nose, mouth, and eyelids; others are sexually transmitted. Our skin protects us in a significant way, and although virus particles on our hands cannot enter our bodies directly, they can easily be transferred to the nose, mouth, and eyes as we touch our faces (thus the admonition to wash hands well and often). And, of course, if we are in close contact with an infected person, we can inhale droplets of virus particles that they exhale.

When a virus enters the body it invades a cell, takes it over, and uses that cell's mechanisms to replicate, grow, and spread to other cells. You have no doubt read a lot about viral load in COVID-19 coverage: for example, that patients with a high viral load tend to get sicker than those with a low viral load. Viral load refers to how much virus is present in an organism. It is determined by measuring the number of copies of the virus present in a millilitre of blood.

Our immediate immune response to a virus, known as the "innate immune response," is to notify surrounding cells of viral activity. This early response is limited, the virus keeps replicating, and the viral load is high just before the onset of symptoms: this is the time when you are contagious and you don't yet know it.

However, this is also the time when the second phase of our immune system kicks in, about 10 to 14 days after exposure. This is the "adaptive" phase of the immune response, when a variety of cells—including T cells and large white blood cells called macrophages—work to kill the virus. Macrophages are sort of like the Pac-Man of the immune system, gobbling up viral invaders at every turn. In this second phase, B cells are also stimulated to make various antibodies that are specifically targeted to kill the particular invading virus.

Blood tests look for IgM antibodies, which are the first to be produced by the B cells. These antibodies are produced relatively early after infection and have only a short-term effect. The second type of antibody, IgG, is produced slightly later, is longer lasting, and should prevent reinfection. Still not clear is how much of each antibody we produce and what minimal amount is needed for protection from a second infection. The research continues and the need for global collaboration is so important.

A doctor from Yale School of Medicine has described the immune system as an orchestra, with an array of cells and various chemicals working in concert. Different cells and different bodily mechanisms have different parts to play in the immune system, like a beautifully orchestrated symphony. We need that symphony in our body, that balanced harmony and ongoing protective effort from our immune system.

Vaccines You Need as a Healthy Adult Woman
Tetanus, diphtheria

You need this vaccine every 10 years, and the next time you get it you should combine it with the vaccine against pertussis, the cause of whooping cough. We have learned that about 20 percent of adults with chronic persistent coughing may have disease related to pertussis because the antibodies we developed if we had the disease as children don't last a lifetime.

Anyone who spends time around babies—and that means grandparents, caregivers, nurses, friends, and young parents—should be immunized because babies under 6 months of age are particularly vulnerable to pertussis. You may be thinking this is a bit extreme because most babies get immunized at 2 months, 4 months, and 6 months. That is true, but it takes time for them to develop immunity. There was an outbreak of pertussis in Los Angeles in 2010, and 10 otherwise healthy, immunized infants succumbed and died of the disease. After this outbreak, the North American guidelines—both those of the U.S. Centers for Disease Control and Prevention and of Health Canada—became much more stringent in an effort to protect the very young.

Pregnant women are now advised to be immunized in their third trimester as this will give the fetus passive antibodies that will help protect the child in its first critical months of life. Because there have been worrisome outbreaks of pertussis, both the U.S. and Canadian guidelines are to immunize with every pregnancy. If you are pregnant or plan to be pregnant, check with your doctor—guidelines are frequently reviewed and updated as information evolves, and you want to make sure you have the benefit of the latest research.

Shingles vaccine

Fifty percent of us will get a case of shingles if we live until we are 80 years old. That's one in two Canadians. The chicken pox virus, called varicella, is living in your nerves, in an area called the dorsal route ganglia. It has been there since you were really young with that typical case of chicken pox—a blistering rash, fever, and an overall feeling of malaise. For years and years your immune system keeps the virus inactive or latent; you might think of it as parked away and forgotten. But with age, with stress, with other illnesses, your immune system is no longer as vigorous and vigilant as it once was, and that varicella virus re-emerges, coming to the surface and damaging the underlying nerve.

Do we care if you get a mild rash, a few blisters? No, we don't care so much because we know that will get better. But do we care if you get significant nerve pain for the next two to five years ... or even longer? Yes, we care a lot about that.

When young people get shingles, their cases are rarely severe; they usually get a rash that is not accompanied by nerve pain. Their shingles will go away in a week to 10 days with antiviral drugs, and then they are okay again. That's why we do not normally immunize people under age 50 against the shingles virus. But for people over 50, immunization is a smart choice. It doesn't eliminate every case of shingles, but it does reduce your risk of nerve damage and the nerve pain caused by the shingles virus, called postherpetic neuralgia. For some people the nerve damage and pain can be lifelong. And it can be truly excruciating.

We treat the pain, of course, but the many drug options all have side effects and risks, and they are often used in combination, which can exacerbate unwanted reactions. There are multiple visits to the doctor and to pain specialists and to others. So the disability mounts, both from the ongoing pain and from the efforts to control it. And unfortunately, not all of this is manageable. In fact, we have seen suicides due to unbearable nerve pain caused by shingles. And shingles is all too often the life-ending episode for an elderly person with multiple other health issues who is on many different medications.

Many patients believe that shingles is like chicken pox, that once you get shingles you will never get it again. Unfortunately that is a misconception: shingles can recur, and it does. So yes, if you are over 50 you should be immunized. And so should your elderly relatives. There are now two vaccines on the market to prevent shingles. The first, a single-shot live virus vaccine called Zostavax, was launched in 2010. It provides reasonably good immunity for the first five to seven years and is more effective in the population between ages 50 and 70 than in the older population. It also decreases the risk of postherpetic neuralgia, a common complication of shingles, by about two-thirds in all ages.

A newer and more robust vaccine called Shingrix requires two shots administered about eight weeks apart. Because this is not a live virus vaccine, it is safer for those who have some level of immune compromise. This vaccine has remarkable efficacy in the general population over the age of 50: it prevents shingles more than 95 percent of the time. Also really special is that there is no reduction of response in older people—because of the design of the vaccine, it elicits a significant response despite age, frailty, and the normal waning of the immune system. So yes, be vaccinated. Yes, I would now recommend the Shingrix vaccine, as did the major guidelines in both the U.S. and Canada. And yes, keep your underlying health robust and free from vaccine-preventable diseases. And finally, yes, be ready for the likelihood of new vaccines with the emergence of new and potentially deadly viruses.

HPV vaccine

The HPV vaccine is an important option for protecting yourself if you are at risk. It decreases your risk of cervical cancer, anal cancer, oral cancers, and recurrence of the cervical cancer that you may have had years ago. HPV infection is very common in adults, and most of us clear the virus easily. But for some there is persistent HPV, and that is what alters cells and leads to cancers. Since we don't know who will clear the virus and who will have persistence, the advice is to immunize, ideally at a young age, before exposure. However, there is benefit from vaccinating, no matter what your age.

HPV 9 refers to the nine subtypes that are now included in the vaccine. The Health Canada national guideline recommends that all 9- to 26-year-olds, both female *and* male, be immunized, and many provinces now provide HPV vaccine in the school system. The Canadian guideline also states that for those patients over the age of 26 who are at risk, the vaccine may be offered to both men and women. There is no upper age limit. If you are 35, 40, 50, whatever, and still potentially exposed, which means sexually active with new partners, there is a benefit to vaccination. We know that cervical cancer peaks for young women in their 30s and 40s, but there is also a second peak in women in their 70s. (A quick note: The official language of Health Canada is that the vaccine "may" be offered; my clinical judgment is that all at-risk individuals should be immunized.)

The research also shows that if you have had an HPV-related disease, such as cervical cancer, now treated, immunization significantly reduces the risk of recurrence either at the same site, such as the cervix, or at another site, such as the vagina or vulva. That HPV disease you had years ago may, in fact, return. We want to guard against that possibility. We want to prevent the occurrence of cancer.

Should everyone over 26 be immunized? No, not necessarily. But should everyone have this conversation with their primary care provider, be assessed, and be vaccinated if at risk? Yes, absolutely. We can say with certainty that HPV-related cancers are significantly preventable—maybe not 100 percent preventable, but 90 to 95 percent preventable—and those are good odds in my book.

Pneumonia and influenza vaccines
Pneumonia and flu together are the number six cause of death in Canada. Pneumonia is an infection of the lungs that needlessly affects millions of people worldwide each year. A vaccination is the best way to prevent the disease or lower your risk. So let's discuss pneumonia vaccine first and then look at influenza.

Common signs of pneumonia are cough, fever, and trouble breathing. In people of all ages a case of pneumonia can be mild—or it can be fatal. In Canada, only 16.7 percent of adults with chronic medical conditions are immunized against Streptococcus pneumonia, which is a bacterial infection. As a result, there has been a dramatic increase in the number of people who get the disease, and about 1,500 Canadian adults die from it every year. Others die from viral forms of pneumonia. Many of these deaths could be prevented with vaccines and appropriate treatment, such as antibiotics and antiviral drugs.

Certain people are more likely to become ill with pneumonia, including the following:

- adults 65 years or older
- children younger than 5 years old
- people who have underlying medical conditions (like asthma, diabetes, or heart disease)
- people who smoke cigarettes
- people whose immune systems are suppressed by diseases such as HIV, leukemia, and other cancers

Pneumonia recommendations for older adults

Pneumonia can be fatal, and before antibiotics it often was. It can be particularly devastating for older adults, and that is partly why two vaccines have been developed for adults; inoculation guidelines are evolving in both the United States and Canada. The current recommendation is that all adults 65 years of age or older who have not previously received the vaccine consider one dose of PCV13; following initial vaccination, they should get a dose of PPSV23 eight weeks later. Both doses are needed to provide maximum protection.

Why two vaccines? Well, partly because the two vaccines contain different subtypes, and stimulate our bodies to produce different types of antibodies. We want the best of both worlds, and to get the best we need to use both vaccines.

Both the U.S. and Canadian medical authorities agree that being age 65 is reason enough to be immunized, even if you are in good health. People with chronic diseases, underlying immune issues, and so on, may be advised to seek immunization at a younger age.

When someone has pneumonia they are more at risk for triggering dysfunction in other organ systems. For instance, we see an increase in heart attacks after pneumonia and worsening of other diseases that may have been stable. Especially for someone whose health is stable only because they are managing one or more chronic diseases well, pneumonia can be a trigger to poorer health outcomes, decreased stamina, and increased frailty, and that may be lifelong. In fact, a respiratory specialist who is a colleague of mine has taught me and countless patients of his simple understanding about pneumonia: "If you get pneumonia, it's simple, you will never be the same."

What you can do to prevent pneumonia and influenza
The popular website **www.health.com** proposes the following practical steps for preventing pneumonia:

- Encourage friends and loved ones with certain health conditions, like diabetes and asthma, to get vaccinated.
- Make sure your children get vaccinated.
- Practise good hygiene; wash your hands regularly or use alcohol-based hand sanitizers.
- Don't smoke.

- Keep your immune system strong—get enough sleep, exercise regularly, and eat a healthy diet.

Okay, so what about flu? Well, the flu vaccine is the only vaccine that changes year by year and needs to be administered every year. The vaccine is produced once the World Health Organization publishes its prediction of which subtypes of influenza are likely to be the worst culprits, based on the flu season in the southern hemisphere, which precedes the flu season here in North America.

There are many kinds of influenza vaccine, and getting one does not prevent every episode of flu. As I mentioned above, in adults a vaccine decreases the severity of disease but does not necessarily prevent the disease entirely. So you may still get the flu despite a flu shot. But you are not likely to be hospitalized and put on a ventilator and die from influenza; neither are you likely to contract pneumonia as a complication of the flu and trigger a serious deterioration of your overall health.

There are many decisions to make in choosing the appropriate flu vaccine for a specific individual because there are many different kinds of vaccines. They come in different doses and they have different delivery systems. For vaccines against viral diseases, there is the further difference between a vaccine with live virus and one in which the virus is attenuated, or inactive. But the biggest difference comes down to this: whether you get vaccinated or do not get vaccinated. Influenza vaccine is an evolving area of research, and my best advice is that you discuss it with your health provider to determine what's right for you.

I remember a slogan from years ago, when John F. Kennedy was running for the U.S. presidency: "Vote for the Kennedy of your choice, but vote!" It's the same thinking here: "Get the influenza vaccine of your choice, but get immunized!" You don't want to end up in emergency, short of breath, feverish, dehydrated, and severely ill. And that really does happen to people all the time. Influenza is not a minor disease: it can take months to recover your energy, your breathing, your normal function, and your usual level of stamina.

Don't Wait—Vaccinate!

It would be negligent of me not to mention the modern movement against immunization. More and more parents are becoming convinced that it is better for their children to strengthen their immune systems by developing antibodies from diseases themselves rather than from vaccinations. They are wrong! If they had lived several generations ago and witnessed the deaths of children due to the very diseases we now avoid through immunization, they might have a very different view. Our grandmothers never seemed to tire of saying "An ounce of prevention is worth a pound of cure." If only they had had the same preventative arsenal we are so lucky to have today!

And Finally...

I have made the case for immunization and talked about various vaccines, but one of the most important issues around immunization is too often overlooked. That issue is record keeping. What vaccinations have you had and when did you have them? Your family doctor may have a great record of what she has given you to date. But vaccines are often given in an emergency room—for instance, when you need stitches or have had an accident. Perhaps you were seen in a travel clinic where they updated certain vaccines; perhaps you were living away from home for a while, at college or in another country that requires particular vaccines we do not need in Canada; or perhaps you have had vaccines that are not routine. Regardless of what vaccines you've had and why you've had them, your immunization record should be accurate.

But how do you get this information, and then manage it on an ongoing basis? And how do you keep track for your kids or a partner or an elderly parent? In Canada, there is no national vaccine registry, no centralized listing of your vaccine history. Public health agencies vary between provinces and territories, as well as states and countries. In Canada, they may have an immunization record for children, but tracking generally stops when people are over the age of 18. The only way to be sure, to be confident that your immunization information is reliable and up to date, is for you to keep your own record.

Luckily, there is an app that can help you do that. It is called CANImmunize and is downloadable for free. It is currently available in both French and English and is being translated into other languages. You can input your own information as well as your family's data. The app also includes information about when boosters are due. It goes wherever your smartphone goes, so when you travel or change doctors or move to a new location, you take the information with you. If knowledge is power, then CANImmunize empowers you: you will always know what vaccination is needed and when it is needed. And that's what good record keeping is all about!

5

MARKING
MIDDLE AGE

Menopause and After

To state the obvious: menopause is a process, not an event. And to be perfectly clear: menopause is not a disease, does not always need treatment, and does not get "cured." Rather it is a time of transition, with lots of changes in a woman's body, not unlike the changes we understand as normal during puberty. It begins with a decline in estrogen production that ultimately results in cessation of ovulation, but a woman's last period is by no means the end of the process. She still has a lot of adjustments to make.

Like It or Not, Menopause Can Feel Like This: The Symptoms ...

The main symptoms of menopause are a reflection of hormonal changes, most notably declining levels of estrogen.

These include mood swings, hot flashes, night sweats and other sleep disturbances, joint pain, and changes in bone and vaginal health. Some lucky women go through menopause free of the uncomfortable symptoms we usually associate with it, but they are probably fewer than 10 percent. Let me remind you of the variation in women's reactions to the hormone changes in pregnancy. Some women get severe nausea and vomiting and feel very unwell, while others don't even know they are pregnant! We all react differently to hormonal fluctuations, and not every woman feels or suffers with every symptom of menopause.

In addition to the end of menstruation, which happens to every woman, most women do have other symptoms, some of which usually go away over time. Hot flashes, for instance. They tend to occur around the transition time, in the first 5 years of menopause, but they also tend to disappear, most of the time beginning to diminish within 3 to 5 years after they begin. Night sweats also tend to resolve with time. I should note here too, though, that approximately 25 percent of women do continue to have hot flashes into their 60s and 70s. This symptom varies greatly from woman to woman, in frequency (how many hot flashes), severity (how intense they are), and timing (how long an individual hot flash lasts and how long overall hot flashes will continue). Some women are called "super flashers"; they have hot flashes of unusual severity for the rest of their lives.

Mood swings are a fairly common symptom of menopause, and although they can be disconcerting to a woman and to those close to her, most women weather the ups and downs without serious long-term implications. However, women who have been susceptible to depression and/or anxiety at times of hormonal instability are, not surprisingly, also vulnerable at menopause. So those women who had trouble with depression around adolescence, or who had postpartum depression, often also have symptoms around menopause. If you are one of them, remain vigilant about the onset of depression/anxiety, and if it does occur I urge you to seek treatment without delay.

Another very, very common experience of menopausal and postmenopausal women is a major change in their libido, which, like other symptoms of menopause, results from the lack of estrogen. Women often tell me they have less interest in sex, they don't feel the same, they don't function the same, and they think things like "It's all over for me."

I think it is very important when you look at something like the Masters and Johnson model of sexual function, which envisions a start, a peak, and a finish to sexual activity, that you realize that process may be true in younger women and it may be true in men but it is not true in menopausal women. Interestingly, a Vancouver-based researcher named Rosemary Basson proposed a different reality, one that has become well accepted in the medical community. Based on her research, first published in 2001, she has created a schematic diagram illustrating sexual function in women as they age, and that diagram portrays sexual experience not as a line with a start and a finish but rather as a circle.

Her research shows that, with menopause, women often lose interest in *initiating* sexual activity; however, if they are intimate, if they are close with their partner and the partner begins sexual activity, they are able to derive pleasure from it. I think her model is much more accurate with regard to how women function simply because I know that a lot of the women in my practice feel this way. But many women, because they have lost interest in initiating sexual activity, and because the idea of sex doesn't have the same appeal, often say, "No way. Why bother?"

When I talk to women in my practice about sexual issues they often respond with a huge sigh of relief. Women tend to think it's a completely personal problem; they think it's just about them or about their partner or their relationship. So it's extremely reassuring for them to learn about Basson's research. (See Chapter 8 for a full discussion of women's sexual health.)

One menopausal symptom that does not go away with time is the genitourinary syndrome of menopause (GSM). Previously referred to as vaginal atrophy, GSM is a medically more accurate term as it covers a broad range of symptoms, not just vaginal atrophy itself. So, what is it? Because of lack of estrogen, the vagina gets dryer and the back wall of the bladder loses its estrogen support. This results in vaginal symptoms like dryness, burning, and itching; it also causes bladder symptoms such as loss of control and results in an increased risk of bladder infections.

It used to be thought that it was not important to treat genitourinary syndrome if a woman was not sexually active, but we realize now that because urinary function is compromised as well, treatment is often warranted. Whether to treat genitourinary syndrome is a personal decision, including whether to treat with a vaginal hormone if dryness is the only symptom. Some women are comfortable with non-estrogen lubricants and moisturizers, but both of these categories of products, though available without a prescription, may have side effects and cause irritation or infection. For example, they may cause the vaginal tissue to become more than normally alkaline, which can promote bacterial overgrowth. They may also promote other chemical alterations. I encourage my patients to consider local estrogen treatment as it has many benefits and very few significant concerns. However, as with any medical intervention, you should discuss this with your doctor. Women should be aware, though, that vaginal dryness gets worse, not better, as they continue to age.

Don't get me wrong: estrogen is not a panacea; it does not solve everything. Adding back estrogen does not necessarily replace lost interest or replace the physiological response so that it is the same as when you were 30. But adding back estrogen can lubricate and make you more comfortable, and for many women it is discomfort that convinces them they are past the time when sex can be good, can be enjoyable for them.

Two other problems occur frequently after menopause. One is that women develop more cardiac complications. Estrogen is protective of the arteries, and that is one reason that women usually get heart disease about 10 years later than men. Before menopause, because their arteries are getting support from estrogen, women generally have less plaque build-up and less endothelial dysfunction (problems with the thin lining of the arteries). With the loss of estrogen through menopause, there can be rapid changes that then catch women up to men vis-à-vis cardiac health. More on heart health in Chapter 6.

The other problem is loss of bone. Estrogen is a prime supporter of bone, and therefore loss of bone strength is a very common result of menopause. And as if that weren't bad enough, loss of bone often happens without any noticeable symptoms. I say often without noticeable symptoms because we generally do not notice that bone strength is being compromised until there is a fracture or until a significant decrease in height has already occurred; these are the two most common events that alert us to the fact that we are at risk for osteoporosis. More on bone health in Chapter 7.

If you are thinking menopause sounds as though it can be just awful, you should be aware that there are effective treatments to relieve some of the most troublesome symptoms. What are the treatments, and how do you decide whether they are appropriate for you? The next section should help answer those questions.

... But It Doesn't Have to Feel That Bad: The Treatments

If you are considering treatment for menopausal symptoms, you should be aware that there are two main categories of treatment—non-hormonal and hormonal—and there are important differences between them.

Non-hormonal treatments

Some of the non-hormonal treatments are absolutely of benefit, particularly for women who either are at risk of developing breast cancer or cannot take hormones because they have had breast cancer. These therapies may also be a choice for a woman who is at risk for blood clots and who therefore must avoid added hormones. One class of non-hormonal drugs that has proven effective is antidepressants. These drugs help control the mood swings of menopause, they help control temperature, and they may help control hot flashes. Most of these benefits were seen as side effects of antidepressants, but now these drugs are routinely prescribed specifically to control the symptoms of menopause. Interestingly, this has become a fascinating, ongoing area of research. In addition, some anti-seizure medications are now being used to control severe hot flashes for women who cannot take estrogen.

However, not all non-hormonal treatments are created equal. Most of the studies done on herbal remedies, soy-based products, and some of the custom-compounded products that we used to call bio-identicals do not show that these confer any benefit. The reality is that most of these products are not medically tested and are not approved by Health Canada or by the FDA as medications, so there is very little reliable research evidence, if any, for their efficacy. Following the guidelines of the Society of Obstetricians and Gynecologists of Canada, I do not routinely use them in my practice.

Hormonal treatments

A woman who does not need to avoid estrogen can turn to one of two types of hormone therapy: *systemic estrogen,* which is the number one treatment for significant, disabling symptoms of menopause (as opposed to symptoms that a woman may simply be aware of as a nuisance but which she is coping with well); and *local estrogen,* which is the treatment of choice if a woman experiences only symptoms that are vaginal and urinary.

Note that this therapy used to be called *hormone replacement therapy (HRT)* but is now called simply *hormone therapy (HT)* or *menopausal hormone therapy (MHT)* because it does not actually replace estrogen at the level at which it was naturally produced before menopause.

Many women who are already on birth control pills at menopause want to stay on them because they feel so well, but I encourage them to begin hormone therapy instead. They are often under the impression that hormone therapy means taking a much higher dose of estrogen than what is in their pill, but it is actually a much lower dose. In fact, the amount of estrogen in current hormone therapy is about one-quarter the dose of estrogen contained in a low-dose birth control pill. The birth control pill has to have a relatively high dose in order to suppress ovulation, but because the ovaries have already shut off due to menopause we can use a much lower dose and still control symptoms effectively.

So yes, hormone therapy is effective in treating menopause symptoms, but there are still decisions to make about how it is delivered, either through systemic delivery or localized delivery. What are some of the considerations in determining which to use?

Systemic estrogen

Depending on which symptoms you're treating and a woman's underlying risk profile, if the decision is to use systemic estrogen you might choose either an oral estrogen or a transdermal estrogen. Oral estrogen comes in pill form, as the term implies, while transdermal estrogen, which enters the blood stream though the skin, comes in many forms—skin patch, gel, cream, and spray. As you can see, there are many choices in making a decision about hormone therapy.

If a woman has an intact uterus (she has not had a hysterectomy) and is on oral estrogen, she also absolutely needs to be on progesterone or another drug to balance the effect of the estrogen on the uterine lining, the endometrium. We now have a new category of medication called a TSEC. A TSEC is a Tissue Selective Estrogen Complex. Basically this is a combination medication of estrogen and a selective estrogen receptor modulator (SERM), a drug that blocks the effect of estrogen in certain tissues, by blocking the estrogen receptor. The estrogen effect has an impact where needed—for example, in diminishing hot flashes. However, in the lining of the uterus, where estrogen can overstimulate the tissue, the SERM blocks that negative effect. The result is that a patient can be on estrogen as part of this TSEC and be protected without the use of progesterone. This class of medication is exciting as we as physicians are able to offer more choices and more individualized options to our patients. The SERM drug not only is effective in treating menopausal symptoms but also has a desired effect on the breast. Estrogen and progesterone can stimulate breast tissue, but the estrogen/SERM combination does not. This is very reassuring: in studies of women on TSECs who were followed up with serial mammograms, we see no change in breast density. The SERM effect is to block the estrogen receptor in the breast, thus blocking tissue stimulation. And SERMs do this in a powerful way.

Tamoxifen is a SERM that is familiar to many of us. It is used in women with breast cancer after they have had surgery to remove the localized cancer. Tamoxifen continues to block the estrogen receptor in the breast, presumably by blocking the tumour cells from estrogen stimulation.

Therefore, it is reasonable to see the benefits of a TSEC— the SERM plus estrogen. It is a great choice for women who need menopausal hormone therapy for hot flashes and night sweats but who clearly do not want the breast stimulation and the increased risk it perhaps brings.

An exciting recent development in treating menopausal symptoms is that an effective medication called a selective tissue estrogenic activity regulator (STEAR) is newly available in Canada. The drug is called tibolone, and although new to North America, it has been available in Europe and other countries since 1988. Tibolone has a unique mode of action: it has estrogenic activity as well as progestogenic and androgenic activity. This means it acts like estrogen, like progesterone, and a little like testosterone. This combination reduces hot flashes and supports bone with minimal risk to breast tissue and the uterine lining. So it is somewhat similar to SERMs, in that it acts like estrogen in some tissue; however, it blocks estrogen or has little effect in other types of tissue.

Also really compelling is that the androgenic activity, or that small amount of testosterone-like stimulus, seems to have a positive impact on both sexual function and reduction of midlife spread (weight gain around the middle). So, while tibolone is clearly indicated for reduction of hot flashes in women who are more than one year past their last cycle, a given patient may find additional benefits from this particular medication.

Oral estrogen is metabolized in the liver, and taking it does increase the risk of blood clots very slightly, which obviously must be considered when deciding the course of treatment. However, for women who experience severe depression due to menopause, oral estrogen has been shown to be more effective than transdermal estrogen in relieving their depressive symptoms. As is so often the case with medical decisions, you have to weigh carefully the potential benefits and the potential harm.

Transdermal estrogen is not metabolized by the liver; it goes right into the bloodstream, and because it bypasses the liver it does not affect a factor called C-reactive protein. There is some research that suggests that therefore transdermal estrogen does not increase the risk of developing blood clots, and that is obviously one of the reasons for choosing a transdermal estrogen for a woman who may be at higher risk of blood clots.

So the first decision is: systemic estrogen, yes or no? If yes, then the decision becomes should it be oral or transdermal? And finally, which product should be used and at what dose? Some doctors may prescribe a higher dose at the start because a woman's symptoms are unbearably uncomfortable, and then, once the symptoms are under control, they may lower the dose. Other doctors may start with the lowest possible dose and increase the dosage as needed until symptoms abate. Both ways are considered acceptable—it really depends on the patient's symptoms and risk profile and the doctor's approach.

That is the art and not the science of medicine. In my own practice, I use both treatment options depending on the patient's history and the particular symptoms we are treating.

Local estrogen

When I talk about local estrogen, I am usually referring to estrogen that is used vaginally, not orally. It may be a cream, a tablet, or an estrogen-infused rubber ring designed to stay in place for three months as the vaginal tissue slowly absorbs the hormone. These treatments are considered local because they are poorly absorbed into the bloodstream. Hence their effects are primarily on the vaginal wall and the back wall of the bladder.

Local estrogen can safely be used twice per week. It lubricates the vagina, supports the delicate tissue, and has a major impact on comfort, on the ability to function sexually, and on the normal maintenance of urinary function and control. There is very little downside, again because it is local treatment. So no, it will not help hot flashes or mood, but yes, you will lubricate more normally with intercourse.

Recently, a newer medication was introduced for the treatment of local vaginal symptoms. Ospemifene is a SERM that is taken orally but has a local effect only on the vaginal tissues, most specifically on the vaginal epithelium, or lining, where it acts like estrogen. It supports the vaginal walls and tissues, resulting in decreased pain and discomfort for women during sexual intercourse. It has a unique tissue profile as a SERM in that it is estrogenic on the vulvar and vaginal tissues and on bone, neutral on the endometrium, and anti-estrogenic in breast tissue. It was FDA approved for treatment of moderate to severe dyspareunia, or pain with intercourse, in

2013, and more recently for vulvar and/or vaginal dryness, which are often symptoms of vulvar and vaginal atrophy (VVA) due to menopause. *Approval in Canada is pending but exciting since this is a choice for women in menopause with sexual issues related to vaginal distress.*

Women often feel itching, dryness, and burning when the vaginal walls are too thin and atrophic, so even if you are not sexually active, local treatment may help you feel more comfortable in your own skin. However, I think it is really important to have reasonable expectations. Yes, sexual function is improved when one is not sore, in pain, or too dry. But this is not a treatment designed to improve libido or sexual desire. Rather, with intimacy and greater comfort and lubrication, there will be an overall improvement in function. And that can't help but improve the situation.

Timing of Estrogen Therapy

When is the best time to begin hormone therapy? This question has basically spurred the creation of a new industry: billions of research dollars have been allocated to come up with a definitive answer.

A study published in 2002 by the Women's Health Initiative (sponsored by the National Institutes of Health in the United States) looked at the effects of estrogen therapy on a large group of women whose average age was 63. The study concluded that estrogen increased the risk of heart attack for women in this group. However, it did not take into account the protective effect of estrogen on the arteries (remember from above that estrogen helps prevent plaque build-up in the arteries). What actually happened is that, because many of these women started on estrogen some 13 to 15 years after menopause, plaque had already begun to clog their arteries; when estrogen was added back for the study it destabilized that plaque, and this impacted heart risk. In addition, many of the study participants already had risk of underlying heart disease: more than 50 percent were smokers, and more than 50 percent were obese or overweight.

What we learned 10 years later in a study called KEEPS (KRONOS Early Estrogen Prevention Study, 2012) is that by adding estrogen around the time of menopause, say between ages 50 and 55, you actually do not increase heart attack risk, and some research suggests you may actually decrease risk in the long run. So if you consider these two studies together, the conclusion is that there are benefits to adding estrogen early and there is risk to adding it late.

What does this mean practically? Well, if I have a patient who is 50 or 51, in good health, with multiple significant menopausal symptoms, I have very little concern about putting her on estrogen. However, if a woman in her mid-60s comes to me with similar symptoms, my medical opinion is that it's too late—I'm not going to put her on estrogen.

Two cases in point. Number one: I had a healthy patient who came to me when she had been in menopause for two years; she was a tennis player, she had never smoked, her cardiac risk in general was low, and she had tried various over-the-counter products but they did not really help. And now she was not sleeping, she was uncomfortable with her husband with regard to sexual function, she was having hot flashes every day and night sweats every night. Was systemic estrogen right for her? My view was that her risk in the next 5 and probably 10 years was very, very low, and we made the therapeutic decision that starting her on hormone therapy was appropriate.

Number two: A 66-year-old woman came into my office and said words to this effect: "I just can't stand it anymore. I was on estrogen for two years when I was in my 50s, but I've been off it since 2002 because I was afraid of the results of that study. I have no sexual interest, my skin is changing, my hair is changing. I'm still getting hot flashes. I still wake up drenched at night. I felt so much better back then, and I really want to go back on estrogen. Can I start hormone therapy again?" I felt a great deal of compassion for this woman, whose symptoms really were disrupting her life, but I had to decline her request to start hormone therapy again because her risk would have been too high. We looked for alternatives, including non-hormonal prescription medications.

The timing hypothesis, then, is simply that there is a window of opportunity when the lining of the blood vessels is relatively healthy and when estrogen may prolong that good health. But later in life, when lack of estrogen has allowed arterial health to decline, it's too late to add back estrogen.

Time from menopause is probably even more important than absolute age in determining whether estrogen therapy is appropriate. You want the time from menopause to be short in order for estrogen to have a positive overall impact and especially not to have a negative impact on the blood vessels.

One of the newest concepts we are discussing in menopause is the concept of cardiovascular age. And this is not the same as cardiac risk. Cardiovascular age can be calculated by looking at a series of factors such as age, gender, weight, height, ethnic group, smoking history, cholesterol level, blood pressure, family history, and a review of chronic medical conditions (including rheumatoid arthritis, chronic kidney disease, atrial fibrillation, and diabetes). A 60-year-old may have a heart age of 40 or 70 depending on these specific factors. It is clear that chronological age alone is not an indicator of heart age.

A heart age of 70 or above is generally a contraindication to hormone use, while a heart age of 60 and below appears reassuring in considering the use of hormones; a heart age between 61 and 69 is likely reassuring as well but warrants careful evaluation.

You can calculate your cardiovascular risk on various websites, including heartage.me, whose assessment tool was launched in concert with the World Heart Federation. But this is an ongoing discussion that needs a personalized approach, so it is something you should talk about with your doctor.

How Long Should I Stay on Hormone Therapy?

One question that women inevitably ask me—and I'm glad they do—is how long they will need to be on hormone therapy if they decide to start it. And, unfortunately, my answer does not always satisfy them because the duration of treatment is different from one woman to the next.

The guideline of the Society of Obstetricians and Gynaecologists of Canada used to be "the lowest dose for the shortest time." The current guideline, however, recommends that treatment should continue while symptoms need treatment. And so for some women treatment may be months but for others it may be years.

What about women who have been on hormone therapy for a prolonged period of time? The North American Menopause Society guidelines suggest that women who have been on long-term treatment and are symptomatic may in fact do well to continue treatment indefinitely. I would not start someone on hormone therapy at age 63, but if she has been on estrogen since age 50 I may continue her on it for the rest of her life if necessary.

Let's review the risks, for with any medication there is always a risk/benefit profile. We know that systemic hormone therapy, though widely used and studied, is not the best choice for everyone. Because it causes a hormone alteration, similar to birth control pills and pregnancy, there is a small increased risk of blood clots, which can mean a blood clot in the legs, a stroke, or a heart attack. These risks are small and considered rare (less than 1 to 10 / 10,000) by the World Health Organization. However, we know that anyone who experiences migraine headaches with aura or who has a history of blood clots, TIAs (transient ischemic attacks), or other related episodes should not take hormone therapy.

There is also thought to be a very small risk in the incidence of breast cancer. This was noted on the Women's Health Initiative study in the estrogen and progesterone group and was not noted in the estrogen-only group. If anything, the estrogen-only group had a decreased risk of breast cancer overall. So it depends on which hormone, for how long, and at what dose. And most recently, a Finnish study concluded that

> the age at HT initiation, regardless whether ET [estrogen therapy] or EPT [estrogen-progesterone therapy], showed no association with breast cancer mortality. In the Finnish unselected population, breast cancer is fatal in one of ten patients. Our data imply that this risk is prevalent in one of 20 patients with history of HT use. This is an important message for women considering or already using HT.

Because this issue is complex and risk may increase with the length of time a patient chooses hormone therapy, it is an area to review every year when the prescription, the need for therapy, and the changing landscape of age and other risk factors are reevaluated.

A Time to Take Stock

I think menopause is an incredible marker in time. It's a time for a woman to review her general health, her lifestyle habits, her symptoms, and her abilities. There are no longer the same family demands and often (thankfully!) there is a renewed focus on her health. She is no longer the very last on her list.

I like to encourage my patients to have a preventative health review at this time. Do you still need contraception? What are the best preventative health care screening manoeuvres that are now recommended, such as colon cancer screening, screening for proper skin care and sun protection, and breast cancer screening? What is the evidence for each option and what is no longer effective? (For example, we no longer do routine chest X-rays for screening, even in long-time smokers.) Evidence evolves and medical practices need to be updated. So when I suggest you speak to your primary health care provider, the goal is for you to receive personalized medicine: What is right for you at your age and stage, with your family history and your individual risk assessment? This is what is required. Remember, you are part of your health care team, and you need to be as informed as possible for that "team meeting."

6

HAPPY VALENTINE'S DAY

Maintaining Heart Health

W ould you believe me if I told you that you can add 14 vital, healthy years to your life? Well, it's true. And you can do it simply by making some of the wise lifestyle choices we have already discussed. Yes—maintaining a healthy lifestyle can delay the onset of heart disease or stroke by as much as 14 years. So says the Heart and Stroke Foundation of Canada, and they should know: they keep track of all the latest research. Just think how much joy 14 healthy, active years can add to your life!

In our society we still tend to think of heart disease as a disease that affects men more than women. The reality, though, is that more women than men die of heart disease every year. Why is that so? And what can we do about it?

Why Do So Many Women
Die of Heart Disease? ...

One factor in the large number of female deaths from heart disease is that women often experience symptoms that are subtly different from the symptoms men experience or that are simply not recognized as cardiac symptoms. Most of the research on heart disease has been done on men (although, thankfully, this is now changing), and therefore doctors are more familiar with men's symptoms. Add to that the fact that the symptoms of heart attack (what you feel, such as chest pressure and fatigue) are often much more subtle in women. And finally, in the absence of known risk factors such as a family history of heart problems, high blood pressure, or high cholesterol, doctors usually rely on the typical risk profile that suggests they should focus only on men over 45 and women over 55 for potential heart disease. But 55 is simply not early enough. We need to pay close attention so that we are sure to identify cardiac risk earlier.

Don't get me wrong: we have made a great deal of progress on heart disease ... in general. Over the past 60 years the number of deaths related to cardiovascular disease has declined by 75 percent. Still, though, every seven minutes someone in Canada has a heart attack, and heart disease and stroke remain among the leading causes of death and hospitalization for both women and men. The result is that many people in our aging population have survived a heart attack and now have ongoing heart disease that limits their activity and their life choices.

The reduction in the number of deaths is related to advances in surgical procedures, drug therapies, and preventative efforts, but the underlying behaviours that lead to heart disease remain unchecked. According to the Heart and Stroke Foundation of Canada, 80 percent of premature heart disease and stroke is preventable by adopting a healthy lifestyle. Yet obesity is on the rise, and with it the prevalence of chronic illnesses such as diabetes and hypertension. The sedentary lifestyle is all too common: many of us sit at a desk all day long; even more of us are addicted to our electronic screens, whether TV or computer or cell phone; and as a population we are much less physically active than our parents or grandparents were. In addition, while once very few women smoked, over the past several generations more and more women have picked up the habit.

... And What Can We Do About It?

The first step in heart health is determining your cardiovascular risk, and there are many ways to do this. One way is by calculating your Framingham Risk Score (FRS). This is a measure of risk that takes into account your age, gender, total cholesterol levels (LDL and HDL), smoking status, and blood pressure, and whether you have diabetes. (If you do have diabetes, the Framingham assessment automatically puts you in the high-risk category, regardless of your other scores.)

Framingham is a town in Massachusetts that was the focus of a large-scale, prospective epidemiological study to evaluate the cardiovascular risk of the population. What this means is simply that researchers did initial assessments of people at whatever age they happened to be at the time and then watched them for the next 50 years or so. By doing this they were able to determine the factors that had the greatest impact on heart health in this population. It is from this study that we first understood that smoking and cholesterol—particularly LDL cholesterol—had such an impact on the heart.

The Framingham Risk Score is based on the data from this study and includes assessment of these high-impact factors. This does not mean that other factors do not also have an impact. Family history, for instance, is an important indicator of cardiovascular risk that the FRS did not originally take it into consideration. However, in 2009 the Canadian Cardiovascular Society published an updated set of guidelines in which the standard FRS was modified to include family history. Some other measures of cardiovascular risk are more elaborate than the FRS, but the FRS provides your doctor with a quick, short-hand perspective on the state of your heart and therefore is widely used as a tool for initial assessment.

The best way I can think of to explain how this works is to tell you exactly what I do to assess cardiovascular risk in a patient. First I look at the factors that can be controlled, treated, or modified, such as blood pressure, cholesterol levels, weight, level of physical activity, and whether the patient smokes or has diabetes. I also try to get a good idea of how much stress the patient lives with on a regular basis. Then I look at the major risk factors that, unfortunately, cannot be controlled, including genes, gender, ethnicity, and age.

I have a blood test done to analyze fats in the blood (called lipids). I also have a test done to analyze the amount of sugar (glucose) in the blood, to determine whether diabetes is a problem. I do routine evaluation of blood pressure, weight, and BMI, and I can also test for the presence of CRP (C-reactive protein), which appears to be correlated to heart disease risk and inflammation of the arteries. If the results of these assessments indicate a potential problem, I have the patient undergo an electrocardiogram (ECG) and perhaps a stress test (treadmill test) to determine heart function during exercise. If further assessment is indicated I do other, more comprehensive tests before making a final determination of cardiovascular risk.

The whole point of doing all this is to identify at-risk patients and to intervene so that we can prevent arteriosclerosis (hardening of the arteries) and atherosclerosis (thickening of the walls of the arteries due to deposits of fatty material that cause plaque build-up). Either of these conditions can result in a heart attack or stroke.

One of the hardest things for me as a physician is when I identify someone who is at risk but who simply does not take my cautions seriously. There is one patient I will always remember because her story is so tragic and could have had a much happier ending. She was relatively young, just 48, a hard-working executive, very successful and very focused on her business. She had no time for exercise, she ate on the run, and she had been a smoker in her 20s and 30s but had given it up in her mid-40s. She was slightly overweight, always trying to lose that extra 10 pounds. And her stress level was through the roof: she was a single mother with one son who had serious health issues that not only required time and money to deal with but that also were a constant source of worry. Her business consumed every bit of energy she had left after dealing with her son's problems, and in the previous three years competitive pressures had begun to threaten her market share. Add to these the fact that she had very little social support as she struggled to keep things together at home and in her business, and you have a recipe for disaster.

So it is very clear what her risk factors were: high stress, overweight, lack of physical activity, and a history of smoking. She always told me she would catch up on healthy living later, once her business was on a firmer foundation and life slowed down a bit. And she really believed she would.

Can you guess what happened? She had a sudden, massive heart attack at her desk and died that day. I understood her pressures and her focus. I empathized with her, remembering my own earlier life and how overwhelmed I had felt with the demands of medical school and training and the crazy hours and workload when I was a resident, but I always encouraged her to make changes—for her sake and for the sake of her son. I think on one level she really did understand that change was necessary, but she simply could not manage to shift her priorities.

I hope you're getting my message: we have to make time for ourselves and make our health a priority—at least some of the time—or time runs out.

Modifiable Risks—The Ones You Can Change
High blood pressure

High blood pressure is often called the silent killer because it shows no symptoms until the damage is done. It is the number one risk factor for stroke and a major risk factor for heart disease. Blood pressure (BP) is determined by measuring both systolic and diastolic pressure. Systolic pressure (the first number) is the pressure created in your arteries when your heart contracts, and diastolic pressure (the second number) is the pressure in your arteries when your heart is at rest. The blood pressure numbers refer to milligrams of mercury (mmHG), a standard measurement of pressure. High blood pressure is defined as systolic blood pressure of 140 mmHG or greater, and diastolic pressure of 90mmHg or greater on at least two separate occasions or when on antihypertensive medication. (The shorthand for this reading is simply 140/90.)

Target blood pressure readings change with age and medical issues—for instance, people with diabetes should maintain a BP reading of 110/70—but generally 120/80 is the goal. Depending on your specific circumstances, your physician may have a different goal for you.

If you have high blood pressure, your heart has to work harder than normal to pump blood through the blood vessels. It can cause arteries to become scarred and allow cholesterol, platelets, fats, and plaque to accumulate in the damaged arteries, which over time causes the arteries to narrow. As we age, our arteries naturally harden and become less elastic; this is a natural process, but uncontrolled high blood pressure makes it happen unnaturally fast.

High cholesterol levels

Cholesterol itself is not a bad thing. In fact, it is necessary for healthy functioning of the body. It is produced by the liver and plays an important role in building new cells, insulating nerves, and producing hormones. But cholesterol also enters your body through foods you eat; animal-based foods like milk, eggs, and meat are major sources of dietary cholesterol. Both a high-fat diet and a sedentary lifestyle can affect your cholesterol levels. And that's where the problem starts.

Too much cholesterol in your body is a risk factor for heart disease, but what level of cholesterol is considered high, and how does your doctor determine whether cholesterol-lowering medication is right for you?

In Chapter 1 I discussed "good" cholesterol (high-density lipoprotein, or HDL) and "bad" cholesterol (low-density lipoprotein, or LDL). Ideally you want your HDL level high and your LDL level low. LDL cholesterol is used as the primary target when deciding whether your cholesterol is on target, and target cholesterol levels differ according to risk category. That's why one of the first steps your doctor takes when assessing your cholesterol profile is determining your overall risk. If you are at low risk for heart disease, your LDL levels can be higher than those of a high-risk individual without causing medical concern. The accompanying box explains the relationship between the Framingham Risk Score and acceptable LDL levels.

Cholesterol and the Framingham Risk Score

For individuals with a Framingham Risk Score of less than 10 percent, which is considered low risk, an LDL level of less than 5.0 is considered acceptable. Individuals with a Framingham score of less than 5 percent can have their cholesterol rechecked in 3 to 5 years, while those with a risk score of 5 to 9 percent should have their cholesterol levels repeated yearly.

Framingham Risk Scores between 10 and 19 percent fall into the moderate-risk category. For moderate-risk individuals, the target LDL level is less than 3.5, and cholesterol-lowering medication will usually be prescribed if the level is greater than this. However, cholesterol-lowering medication will also be recommended for moderate-risk individuals if their LDL level is less than 3.5 but they also have elevated levels of a different marker called non-HDL.

Finally, Framingham Risk Scores of 20 percent or greater are considered high risk. All high-risk people should consider treatment with cholesterol-lowering medications, regardless of their LDL cholesterol levels.

We are learning that, in general, lower LDL is better because it lowers your risk of heart disease. I will not be surprised—and you shouldn't be either—if we see that all these numbers, or set points, are lowered as we aim to reduce heart disease risk further. In fact, the newest guidelines continue to set lower limits of LDL, not just in patients with heart disease but also in others in order to prevent them from developing heart disease.

Many of my patients almost despair when we talk about cholesterol because they are already on a low-fat diet with little added cholesterol. But some people have a genetic predisposition for producing excess cholesterol from the liver—no matter how carefully they eat—and so higher than average lipid levels tend to run in some families. For people with this genetic propensity, medication is literally a lifesaver.

For others, who have a less worrisome family history and an overall active lifestyle, it is often sufficient to monitor cholesterol levels and consider medications only as they age.

It is important that we know the cholesterol numbers because they help us determine one aspect of risk, but remember that what we really need to focus on is overall risk assessment. So get your readings, but realize that they do not tell the whole story.

Diabetes

Having diabetes doubles your chances of having a heart attack or stroke, and according to the Canadian Diabetes Association, people with diabetes may develop heart disease 10 to 15 years earlier than those who do not have the disease.

Everyone is aware of diabetes, but a surprisingly small number of people actually know what it is. They know it has something to do with blood sugar levels (the amount of glucose in the blood), and they know that insulin is used to control it. They also know it is a chronic disease and that it can be fatal if not managed properly. But most would be hard-pressed to say more than that. So let's start with a quick explanation, and let's start our explanation with the pancreas and how it functions.

The pancreas is an organ about six inches long that is located at the back of the abdomen, behind the stomach, and it releases hormones into the digestive system. If blood sugar levels get too high, the pancreas releases insulin, a hormone that allows cells to absorb sugar, which can then either be used as energy or stored as fat. The result of this absorption is that blood sugar levels fall again and a healthy glucose level is maintained.

In diabetes, though, one of two things happens: either the pancreas cannot release enough insulin to control blood sugar levels, or the body cannot effectively utilize the insulin it does produce. Whichever mechanism of diabetes is at play, it is problematic because the body needs insulin in order to convert sugar to energy. And the result is the same: glucose levels rise to a point that can cause damage to organs, nerves, and blood vessels.

So there is no question that insulin is a lifesaver for many people with diabetes. Type 1 diabetes usually has an abrupt onset and is characterized by a complete lack of insulin. Type 2 diabetes often is slow in onset with rising glucose levels over time, as the pancreas becomes less and less able to produce enough insulin for the daily needs. While type 1 diabetes is always treated with insulin, type 2 may be initially treated with diet and oral medications, in the effort to decrease the glucose by healthier choices so the pancreas can produce less insulin. The drugs stimulate insulin production or the more effective use of the insulin that is produced. However, in type 2 diabetes, there may be a need for insulin as well, as the pancreas is not able to respond to changing glucose levels. There is no question, though, that making changes in lifestyle can go a long way in controlling diabetes. Depending on a person's situation, weight loss, exercise, and proper diet may reduce the burden on the pancreas and delay the need for medications. This is true even if these lifestyle changes start later in life. Eventually, however, most people with diabetes will need drugs as the pancreas becomes less and less able to produce enough insulin.

Here is one example. An 80-year-old who had diabetes was able to keep the disease in check and delay the need for insulin by swimming three to four times a week and adopting a special diet. In fact, dietary intervention can be so effective that there is actually a medical term based on it: diet-controlled diabetes.

Sometimes, however, the disease is too aggressive and there is an urgent need to start medication immediately. Given that people with diabetes are much more likely to have earlier heart disease, they are automatically classified as high risk when we look at Framingham. So typically there is a need to control glucose, BP, and lipids immediately.

I always recommend that my patients know the symptoms of diabetes and take action immediately if they think they may be at risk. A list of symptoms follows. If you recognize them as applying to you, tell your doctor at the first opportunity.

Symptoms of type 1 diabetes
- Frequent urination
- Excessive thirst
- Increased hunger

- Weight loss
- Tiredness
- Lack of interest and difficulty concentrating
- A tingling sensation or numbness in the hands or feet
- Blurred vision

Symptoms of type 2 diabetes
- Weight gain
- Fatigue
- Overall sluggishness

Stress

When stress is constant, your body remains in high gear on and off for days or weeks at a time, or even for longer. Although there is no linear link between stress and heart disease, stress in itself can be a risk factor for cardiac complications. It causes constant elevation of adrenalin, which puts the body into high gear. We know that continuing high stress levels can worsen other risk factors, such as high blood pressure and high cholesterol, both of which are key contributors to heart disease. In fact, because chronic stress also raises the heart rate, it can lead to high blood pressure even in people who previously had no problem.

Long-term stress can also lead a person to make unhealthy choices. They may feel there just is not enough time to keep up their exercise routine. Or they make turn to "comfort foods" for instant gratification rather than maintaining healthy eating habits—which, in turn, contributes to weight gain, another risk factor for heart disease. One of my central messages is that you have to make yourself a priority, but when you're too stressed out you are not the priority. This may be okay part of the time—for instance, in short-term, urgent situations—but it is not okay if your stress is ongoing and seemingly endless.

Excessive alcohol consumption

There is some evidence that moderate drinkers and those who drink just a little have a somewhat lower risk of heart disease and stroke than those who do not drink at all or who drink excessively. And while the science is not conclusive yet on why this is true for alcohol in general, it is thought that the antioxidants in red wine have a protective effect. However, drinking too much of any type of alcohol can increase your blood pressure and contribute to the development of heart disease and stroke.

So what exactly is moderate drinking? The Heart and Stroke Foundation defines moderate drinking for women as one to two drinks a day most days to a weekly maximum of 10; for men, it's three drinks a day most days to a weekly maximum of 15. I have to smile when some of my patients try to demonstrate that they drink only moderately by saying to me something like this: "Well, Dr. Brown, my husband and I split a bottle of wine at dinner every evening, but that's the only alcohol I drink ... unless we're at party." I smile, but only because it reminds me how few people really understand the word "moderate" as it applies to alcohol. Half a bottle of wine is not quite within the bounds of moderate; it is actually two and a half glasses of wine, not two glasses.

You may be thinking, "Really, Dr. Brown, are you going to quibble over half a glass of wine?" But that extra half a glass can add up, and it adds up to no good. In fact, it might be wise to limit your consumption of alcohol considerably below the weekly maximum of 10 drinks. We know, for example, that drinking more than 7 to 9 drinks per week can increase the risk of breast cancer.

I'm not an abolitionist, and I'm not going to preach abstinence from alcohol, but I will ask you to be careful with your alcohol consumption. Review what you are actually doing when you drink, tally how much you drink in a week—including the weekend BBQ and the girls' night out—and please make sure that your glass is not "Keg-sized."

Guidelines for drink size

One drink means
- 341 mL / 12 oz. (1 bottle) of regular-strength beer (5% alcohol)
- 142 mL / 5 oz. wine (12% alcohol)
- 43 mL / 1 1/2 oz. spirits (40% alcohol)

Source: Heart and Stroke Foundation of Canada

Overweight/obesity

At least 2.8 million people die each year around the world as a result of being overweight or obese. The science is clear: if you are overweight or obese, you are at risk of a heart attack or stroke. Obesity contributes to high blood pressure, glucose intolerance, and type 2 diabetes. In addition, high cholesterol levels from a high-fat diet, combined with little or no exercise, will almost always lead to cardiovascular disease. In Chapter 1 I discuss the importance of maintaining a healthy weight and BMI as important components of healthy aging. Please take that message to heart.

Smoking

Smoking is a major cause of heart disease. It damages the lining of the arteries and puts you at high risk for stroke. End of story! There is no safe lower limit. Even regularly smoking just one or two cigarettes when you are out socially or when you are in a stressful situation increases your risk of heart disease. The risk of various cancers is obviously a major concern with smoking, but so is the ongoing damage to the arteries. If you are a smoker, the most significant impact you can make in your risk profile vis-à-vis heart disease is to stop smoking. Even if that means gaining a bit of weight and feeling more stressed, stopping smoking will give you the greatest bang for your buck in reducing heart disease risk.

Lack of physical activity

You may remember from the discussion of the importance of regular physical activity in Chapter 2 that a sedentary lifestyle is defined as not doing regular physical exercise. Lack of physical activity increases the risk of diabetes and high blood pressure, both of which compromise cardiovascular health, so if you do not exercise you are putting yourself at risk of developing heart disease. I won't repeat here all that I said in Chapter 2 about exercise, but let's remember just how important it really is.

Sleep

Sleep is important for your heart. We know that heart attacks often happen very early in the morning. We know that if people do not get truly restful sleep, if they do not get the normal dip in blood pressure during sleep, they are at greater risk for heart disease later on. If you are concerned because you feel you're not getting enough good-quality sleep, you can review the 10 strategies for better sleep listed in Chapter 2.

Non-Modifiable Risks—The Ones You Cannot Change

Most cardiovascular disease is caused by risk factors that can be controlled, treated, or modified, as just discussed: high blood pressure, high cholesterol levels, diabetes, stress, excessive alcohol consumption, overweight/obesity, smoking, and lack of physical activity. However, there are also major cardiovascular risk factors that cannot be controlled. Your age, gender, ethnicity, and genetic inheritance/family history cannot be modified.

Age

Cardiovascular disease becomes increasingly more common as we age. Even in someone who has no heart disease, the heart undergoes subtle changes with age. One common change is that the relaxation of the heart muscle between beats can become less complete; this results in stiffening of the pumping chambers, which can affect how efficiently they work. Overall, being active and physically fit delays this process.

Gender

According to the World Heart Federation, "the risk of stroke is similar in men and in women, but a man is at greater risk of heart disease than a pre-menopausal woman. Once past menopause, though, a woman's risk is similar to a man's." Fortunately, women can take steps early in adulthood to reduce their risk of heart disease. And understanding the unique symptoms of heart disease in women can literally save lives.

We all worry about breast cancer, and rightly so, but medical statistics reaffirm that heart disease is the number one killer of women in Canada.

Heart attack symptoms for women

A heart attack occurs when the blood supply to the heart muscle is blocked. The most common heart attack symptom is a pain, pressure, or discomfort in the chest, but it is not always severe or even the most prominent symptom. Women are more likely than men to have heart attack symptoms unrelated to chest pain, and sometimes a woman will have a heart attack with no chest pain at all.

When they do have chest pain, women may describe it as pressure or tightness, and they may experience only subtle chest pain. This is because they tend to have blockages not only in their main arteries but also in the smaller arteries that supply blood to the heart—a condition called small vessel heart disease or microvascular disease.

Common heart attack symptoms in women include these:

- Neck, jaw, shoulder, upper back, or abdominal discomfort
- Shortness of breath
- Right arm pain
- Nausea or vomiting
- Sweating
- Light-headed or dizziness
- Unusual fatigue

Mental stress may trigger heart attack symptoms in women, but women's symptoms may occur when they are resting, or even when they are asleep. Because their symptoms are not those typically associated with a heart attack and because women may downplay their symptoms, they tend to show up in emergency rooms after heart damage has already occurred. They may complain of extreme fatigue or weakness in the arms, and all too often they are sent home after being told that they are just anxious. If you experience the symptoms noted in the box or think you are having a heart attack, call for emergency medical help immediately. Don't drive yourself to the emergency room unless you have no other options. Better to be safe, checked out, and discharged than to sit at home, considering your options—and perhaps letting further heart damage occur.

Ethnicity

One individual's cardiovascular risk may be higher than another's simply by virtue of their ethnicity. For example, diabetes is a major risk for heart disease, and people from Southeast Asia are more at risk for diabetes than North American Caucasian people; they also tend to contract it about 10 years earlier. And when compared to white people, black people tend to develop hypertension—another significant risk for heart disease—at a younger age. The bottom line, though, is that no matter your ethnicity, individual assessment is key to protecting your health.

Genetics and family history

A family history of heart disease can also indicate a person's risk. If you have a first-degree blood relative—a parent, sibling, or child—who has coronary heart disease or has had a stroke before the age of 55 (for a male relative) or 65 (for a female relative) the risk increases. If you are at risk because of your family history, I strongly suggest you talk with your doctor and assess your risk factors on an on-going basis.

Strategies to Reduce the Risk of Heart Attack and Stroke

I've already told you I'm biased. As a family doctor, I believe in the power of aggressive prevention: I want to incorporate every manoeuvre, every option, to reduce risk for every patient.

So what do I mean by aggressive prevention? Here is an example. I have a patient who was obese, about 35 to 45 pounds above ideal weight (and by ideal I do not mean thin but rather average). She no longer smoked and drank only moderately but was extremely stressed and too busy to exercise. She had both diabetes and hypertension. I discussed her risk factors with her and made it clear that I could help her only if she wanted to help herself. All the right drugs will help only if you take them properly, and all the right counselling will help only if you act on good advice and make the lifestyle changes that are required to decrease your risk.

My patient was overwhelmed, but I was adamant. I told her that she really had no choice if she wanted to protect her health and increase her chances of living independently into old age. I told her that her obesity, sedentary lifestyle, and constant stress level would kill her, sooner or later … and probably sooner. Sometimes a doctor just has to be blunt to make a patient understand the seriousness of the situation.

I remember saying to her, "I'm not giving up on you unless you give up on you!!!"

Well, long story short, she has now lost 20 pounds and started a walking program. So far, so good. Not miraculous results, not instant results, but this is a marathon, not a sprint. We both feel relieved she is moving in the right direction with her health. And she is taking her medications faithfully and carefully.

When I measure her numbers—glucose, lipids, blood pressure, BMI—everything is moving in the right direction. What a relief … for both of us! She is my poster girl for living athletic and not saying, "OMG, how can I do this?"

Early in the course of heart disease, lifestyle changes may actually trump medications. Does that sound too dramatic? I hope not, because it is true. Medication versus lifestyle—it's not an either-or choice. But certainly many patients have been able to stop taking their medications after beginning a dedicated exercise program and losing weight. It's a wonderful feeling being able to encourage patients to discontinue prescription drugs. But the doctor–patient relationship is a partnership and we both are on the same team, so it's important to realize that lifestyle modifications and medication can complement one another and should be used together when needed.

I hope I've been successful in delivering my message—and enough information for you to take it to heart. If you want to have a significant impact on your heart health, there are actions you can take right now to decrease your cardiovascular risk over the long term. To reiterate:

- Start eating a healthy diet.
- Begin a physical activity routine that includes doing moderate to vigorous aerobic activity for 150 minutes a week. Start walking now!
- If you smoke, become smoke-free.
- If you drink alcohol, drink moderately.
- Get to and maintain a healthy weight.
- Pay attention to your stresses and your lifestyle choices (stress can make poor choices easier!).
- And finally, see your doctor to decide your risk profile and whether you need more attention, more testing, or medications.

It's Time to Give Your Health a Hearty Welcome

I've mentioned before that it's never too early—or too late—to make your own health a priority, so if you have any concerns at all about your heart health, I recommend asking your doctor to conduct a Framingham Risk Score. Understand your numbers and then follow up as required. Just like shopping for a bathing suit, this is *not* a one-size-fits-all scenario.

Life is an exciting journey; let's make it a long and healthy one!

7

ROBUST OR BRITTLE?

Bone Health and
Osteoporosis

I n one way it is chronologically fitting that we discuss bone health near the end of the book because the most severe consequences of poor bone health usually become evident with aging. At the same time, though, one expert on osteoporosis calls it a pediatric disease. If this seems contradictory to you, don't worry—it should soon become clear that it makes a great deal of sense.

It's Alive!

Let's start with a little bit about bone itself. When talking about bones it is important to understand the difference between the terms *micro-architecture* and *bone mass*. Micro-architecture refers to the quality of bone, while *bone mass* describes the quantity of bone. Both are essential to maintaining skeletal integrity; healthy bone has good architecture *and* good mass, and compromised bone can involve deterioration of either of these or of both of them at the same time.

Bone is living tissue that is continuously changing throughout a person's life, just like skin. Various protein fibres and minerals, mostly calcium, together form the bone's structural foundation, which is the micro-architecture mentioned above. This micro-architecture serves the same purpose in bone that strut supports serve on a bridge: it makes bones strong and it makes them flexible. Bone mass, on the other hand, is the total amount of bone. To keep with the bridge analogy, it is all the steel and concrete that goes into the building of a bridge.

Bone density is another important component of bone; it refers to the amount of calcium and other minerals present in a segment of bone. When we measure bone health, we're actually measuring bone density, and the test we do is called a bone mineral density test (discussed later in this chapter).

Many people think of bone as stable and unchanging once we reach adult height, but it is actually dynamic, constantly breaking down and repairing itself through a process called remodelling. Bone-eroding cells called osteoclasts invade the bone's surface, dissolving minerals and causing small cavities in the surface of the bone; at the same time, bone-forming cells called osteoblasts fill in the cavities with new bone until the bone surface is completely restored.

Osteoporosis: When Things Go Wrong

Through remodelling, this healthy, living bone tissue is constantly in a state of balance. Unfortunately, though, interruption of this balance can result in osteoporosis. Many factors can disrupt this balance, and number one among them is age. This is because bone naturally deteriorates with age: as we get older, the cells that erode bone continue to function fairly well, but the activity of the cells that rebuild bone slows down. In other words, the remodelling of bone is no longer balanced. You might think of it this way: you've hired a contractor to renovate your home, the demolition phase is complete and the restoration has begun, but then the contractor disappears to work on another job, so you're left with a house that's only partially remodelled. Although most likely the contractor will reappear to finish the job, without pharmaceutical help the bone-building cells will not.

Osteoporosis Canada describes osteoporosis as "a disease characterized by low bone mass and deterioration of bone tissue. This leads to increased bone fragility and risk of fracture (broken bones), particularly of the hip, spine, wrist and shoulder." I would add, though, that all bones can be affected.

Osteoporosis is more common than many people realize: one in four women will get osteoporosis (usually after menopause), and one in eight men over age 50 will develop the disease. It is a serious disease: if you need to be convinced, just look at the photographs (see Figure 2 on next page).

Figure 2: Normal Bone vs. Osteoporosis

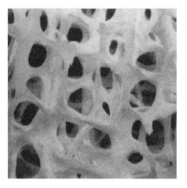 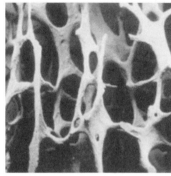

Normal Bone   Osteoporosis

Source: NIH Consensus Development Panel on Osteoporosis. JAMA 2001.

There are two common misconceptions about osteoporosis of which you should be aware. One is that osteoporosis
is exclusively a woman's disease—it is not! The other is that
osteoporosis is a part of normal aging—it is not! In fact, both
men and women suffer from osteoporosis, and although most
people associate it primarily with older adults, it can strike
at any age. Some bone loss does occur naturally with age,
but this is different from the catastrophic, disease-driven loss
caused by osteoporosis.

Sex hormones help to build and maintain bone. When a
woman begins to lose estrogen during menopause, she can
experience bone loss at a rate of 2 to 5 percent per year, which
will increase her risk of developing osteoporosis. That is why
postmenopausal women are at particular risk. Women are
also at increased risk of osteoporosis if they begin menopause

prematurely (either naturally or as a result of surgery), if they have not menstruated for a few cycles (apart from pregnancies), or if they have an ovulation disorder.

Men, on the other hand, lose bone more slowly as they age; their incidence of bone loss normally begins to increase after about age 65. The most common causes of osteoporosis in men younger than 65 are secondary causes, such as use of certain steroids, low levels of testosterone, and excessive alcohol intake. By the time people are in their 80s and 90s, though, the risk is about the same for men and women. And we now know that some commonly used drugs can affect the rate of bone loss as well, such as medications for GERD (gastroesophageal reflux disease) and for depression.

A fracture is often the first indication of trouble

You might think that our main aim in dealing with osteoporosis is to achieve greater bone density, but that is not the case. We know how to improve bone density: we could do it simply by using fluoride, but fluoride results in bone that is as brittle as a china plate and will crack like one. So, yes, we can achieve greater bone density that way, but not greater bone quality.

Our main focus in dealing with osteoporosis is to prevent fracture, and therefore prevention of fracture is the measure of success. The reason that fracture takes centre stage is clear: because too often a fracture is the dramatic event that first indicates a person has osteoporosis.

Let's look at what fracturing a bone means. There are two types of fractures: traumatic fractures and fragility fractures. As its name implies, a traumatic fracture is the result of some forceful trauma to the body. A fragility fracture, on the other hand, happens with either no bodily impact or relatively slight bodily impact. It is defined as a fracture that occurs with minimal trauma as the result of a fall from your standing height or from one to three steps up. For example, if you step off the curb and fracture your ankle, that is considered a fragility fracture; if you fall on the ice and fracture your wrist, that is a fragility fracture; but if you get hit by a truck and fracture any bone, that is a traumatic fracture. Probably eight out of every ten fractures in people over the age of 50 are fragility fractures. Therefore we assume a fracture at that age is a fragility fracture unless it is evident that it was caused by trauma.

With advanced osteoporosis bone becomes so fragile that a person can experience a fragility fracture simply because their body is out of the normal plane of movement, as for instance when a vertebra (or more than one) fractures as the result of a person twisting to look over their shoulder. One surprising finding is that if you fall twice within a year, even if you do not fracture, your risk of fracture increases because if you fall that often you are more likely to continue to fall, and if you keep falling sooner or later a fall will result in a fracture.

When I discuss bone health with my patients, I tell them, "What you want is to bounce, not break, when you fall." But people do break bones. At least one in three women and one in five men will suffer from an osteoporotic fracture during their lifetime, and they will fracture differently at different ages.

With people in their 50s and 60s what we typically see are wrist fractures—they put out their hands to break a fall and they break their wrist. In fact, wrist fractures are the most common type of fracture in women under age 75. When people are in their 60s and 70s we start to see vertebral fractures, which are fractures of the bones of the spine. In their 70s and 80s we start to see hip fractures. Fracturing your wrist in your 50s is an indicator that your bone quality is not as good as it should be and that you are more at risk for fracturing other bones later in life. Your bone density could be still reasonably good, but if you have a fragility fracture of your wrist we know that your bone quality is not as good as it should be.

Hip fractures

The most common sites of fractures are the hip, wrist, spine, and shoulder, as indicated in the Osteoporosis Canada definition of the disease mentioned above. Of these, hip fractures are by far the most devastating.

The stats are startling. Most hip fractures are in people 75 years old or older, and most hip fractures are life-changing events for those who experience them. About 40 percent of people who fracture a hip do not recover their former health and mobility and do not go back to independent living. About

25 percent of women and 37 percent of men who fracture a hip die in the first year after the fracture, and many who survive are permanently disabled. The death rate is high because the older you are the more likely you are to fracture a hip, and the older you are the more likely you are to have chronic diseases. Therefore the hip fracture affects your general health. It makes you sedentary at first and then less mobile for some time afterwards, and this affects your normal breathing—all of which makes it easier for a blood clot to form, which can then result in a pulmonary embolism causing death. All because you fractured your hip.

I'd like to take a minute here to point out that, yes, a hip fracture can be a tragic, life-changing event for the person who fractures, but it can also have devastating consequences for that person's spouse and family. Here is a case in point.

One of my patients came to the office accompanied by her elderly father. I had never met her parents before and asked her why her dad was with her. She said her dad was a big, strong guy and her mother was a little, petite woman, and they had lived together for 60 years in a small house in a small town in Ontario. Her mother took care of the bills, did the banking, did the grocery shopping, sorted and read the mail, read the TV guide, and worked the VCR; her father carried the groceries, shovelled the snow, did the painting and household repairs, etc. But then her mother slipped and fell and broke her hip. She had her hip replaced and went to a rehab centre where initially she was doing really well … until she developed a pulmonary embolism from a blood clot and died.

The ongoing tragedy of the story is that her father had never learned to read, so he could no longer live by himself because he couldn't do the banking, he didn't know what was in the mail, he couldn't make a grocery list, he couldn't even figure out what was on TV unless he resorted to channel flipping. And so even though he was in excellent physical health, he could no longer live independently. He was living with his daughter for a short time until he could transition into a seniors facility. This story illustrates one reason I think we need to be so aggressive about bone health and why we should be so excited about preventative options. Osteoporosis is not only an individual's hip fracture—it can also be a family's tragedy.

Just a quick note: a fragility hip fracture in a younger woman is unusual, and usually there is an explanation—certain drugs and certain genetic factors can compromise the integrity of bone—but in general your risk of fracture simply increases as you age.

Preventing fractures: Diet and exercise, again

So, when do we want to start working hard to prevent osteoporosis from happening? I mentioned in the first paragraph of this chapter that one expert refers to osteoporosis as a pediatric disease. That expert is Dr. Robert Josse, who insists that preventative measures should start in childhood. Not getting enough exercise as a kid, not drinking enough milk as a kid, having too many soft drinks—those kinds of habits in young people have significant long-term negative effects on bone health. Take soft drinks, for instance. They contain phosphate, and phosphate alters the calcium metabolism so that calcium leaks out of bone. So young women who avoid milk and drink diet cola all day may be maintaining a slim figure, but they are not doing themselves any favours with regard to bone strength. The effect of not drinking milk or eating other dairy products should be self-evident: these are the best dietary sources of calcium.

Dietary prevention: Calcium and vitamin D

In order to build and maintain strong bones, we need to mineralize our bones. Easy to say, but is it easy to do? The answer is yes. And part of the answer includes the choices we make about food. Ideally we start in childhood by ingesting sufficient calcium in ways that our bodies can absorb. This helps bones develop well right from the start.

As we age, and whether or not we got enough calcium from our diets earlier in life, we want to keep the bone that we do have strong; we want to continue to mineralize it. I mentioned above that estrogen supports bone health, but with menopause women lose the bone-protective benefit of estrogen. Everyone, no matter what their age, should be careful to get enough calcium, but postmenopausal women especially need to include enough calcium-containing foods in their diet.

As mentioned in Chapter 1, it is better to eat foods that are rich in calcium than it is to take calcium supplements because the calcium from food sources is better absorbed. Milk, cheese, and yogurt are great sources of calcium—remember, you can choose low-fat options!—and they are all better choices than just popping a calcium supplement.

For adults who cannot tolerate dairy, getting calcium from supplements is better than getting no calcium at all. The recommended dose for people over 50 is 1200 mg a day. If you can tolerate dairy, you need the equivalent of one good serving of dairy at each meal. But many people are lactose intolerant and cannot digest dairy products easily. What should they do? The following box lists some recommendations from Osteoporosis Canada. See Section A of the Appendix for a link to Osteoporosis Canada's comprehensive listing of the calcium content of various foods.

Non-Dairy Food Sources of Calcium Recommended by Osteoporosis Canada

- Calcium-fortified soy, almond, and rice beverages (check the nutrition labels)
- Calcium-fortified orange juice (check the nutrition labels)

> • Canned salmon or canned sardines (When you eat the bones that have been softened by the canning process, these foods are excellent sources of calcium.)
>
> *Source: www.osteoporosis.ca/osteoporosis-and-you/nutrition/ calcium-requirements.*

There has been an enormous amount of research on the potential benefits of vitamin D, and one clear conclusion is that it helps in a number of the metabolic pathways that are involved in absorption of calcium into the body. Sunshine is a great natural source of vitamin D, but in North America, even if you spend time out in the sun, two things are operative: (1) the sun provides less vitamin D here because of its angle to the earth, and (2) many people use sunscreen, which blocks absorption of vitamin D from the sun. So, for most of us, being out in the sun is not good enough for absorbing vitamin D. Some research actually suggests vitamin D is more important than calcium for bone health, but most experts maintain that you need both.

New data on vitamin D show that low levels may have a negative effect on the immune system. Specifically, studies of patients with COVID-19 show that those with higher levels of vitamin D had better outcomes than those with low levels.

An article published in May 2020 by Osteoporosis Canada notes that "two recent studies have suggested that low levels of vitamin D may be associated with an increased risk of severe COVID-19 infections." The article also states that researchers "noted that countries with low levels of vitamin D had a higher number of COVID cases, as well as the highest mortality rates from COVID" and "that severe COVID-19 infections appeared to be more common in countries where vitamin D deficiency is more common."

Therefore, although there may be a number of other variables at play, researchers are looking at a possible link between vitamin D deficiency and an impaired immune response to COVID-19. We know already that vitamin D is good for bone health, and we are now investigating whether it also has a significant impact on the immune system generally.

Although I encourage patients to get their calcium from food rather than from calcium supplements, with vitamin D my advice is different: buy vitamin D supplements and take them every day. How much? The recommended dose is 400 to 1000 IUs for adults under 50 and 800 to 2000 IU for adults over 50. This is a must!

Exercise for strength and balance

I said above that the number one aim in dealing with osteoporosis is to prevent fractures. Keeping bones well mineralized is one way to do this—it is the dietary approach. But we also try to prevent fracture by encouraging people to exercise regularly.

As we age, keeping our balance can become more difficult. Strength training helps to maintain good muscle tone, and that is important because strong muscles help maintain balance. Studies of women over the age of 80 in nursing homes have shown that working on upper body strength made it easier for them to transfer from wheelchair to bed. This is a major benefit since many falls—and many fractures—happen in exactly that type of transition.

Exercise also helps to keep the body aligned properly so that we are less likely to fall and more likely to "fall well" if we do; both of these make a fracture less likely. Some exercises are thought to be better than others, and balance exercises are especially important. One type of exercise in particular—tai chi—has been shown to correlate with better balance, which results in reduced risk of falling. And if you don't fall, you are less likely to fracture. You should note, though, that many osteoporosis experts say that any exercise is better than no exercise.

Remember from Chapter 2 that it is never too late to start exercising. And there's always a benefit—obviously the benefit is greater the younger you are when you begin.

Osteoporosis Canada recommends various types of exercises for people who have osteoporosis, including strength training, posture training, balance training, and weight-bearing aerobic activity. See Section B in the Appendix for a link to this information.

Evaluation and Treatment

It's all well and good—and necessary—to talk about and to initiate the preventative strategies of a healthy diet and regular exercise, but is that enough?

Evaluation

Over the years, many women in my practice have asked me how they would know if they were already losing bone. It's a very good question, because osteoporosis is known as a "silent thief"; it is stealthy as it quietly destroys your skeleton. However, there may be warning signs and symptoms of the disease in some individuals. For instance, if you lose more than two centimetres of height in a year or more than four centimetres altogether, have persistent bone pain, spinal deformities, or recurrent fractures or fractures from minimal trauma, you should talk to your family physician about being assessed.

You should also talk to your physician if you answer yes to either of the following two important questions: Have I had a fracture since age 40? Have I fallen since age 40, even without fracturing a bone? Both a previous fracture and a history of falls indicate significant risk for osteoporosis. In fact, falling is one of the factors doctors look at in evaluating whether someone is frail, and frailty itself is a risk for fracture.

Most of the women who have asked me how they would know if they were at risk of fracture had no symptoms at all. Fortunately for them—and for all of us—it is easy for a physician to conduct a fracture risk assessment. A fracture risk assessment evaluates your personal risk, based on your age, your family history, and any known complicating factors such as whether you are on certain medications (especially prednisone) and whether you have certain diseases (such as rheumatoid arthritis).

It also may include a bone mineral density test (BMD), which I mentioned above. This painless test, similar to an Xray, will determine how dense the bone is. In other words, it measures the mineral concentration of the bone—especially how much calcium is present. The hip, the forearm, and the bones of the back are the ones that are most frequently tested.

A BMD can determine not only whether you have osteoporosis but also whether you risk developing it at some future time. Osteoporosis Canada recommends that menopausal women and men aged 50 to 64 with risk factors for fracture should have a BMD done, and that women and men under 50 should also have one done if they have a disease or condition associated with low bone mass or bone loss. And by age 65, everyone—women and men—should have at least one bone density test to evaluate their status and establish a baseline.

Another method for evaluating bone health is called FRAX, which stands for Fracture Risk Assessment Tool. Developed by researchers at the University of Sheffield, FRAX is an evidence-based assessment, with reproducible results. This simple twelve-point questionnaire calculates the percentage risk of suffering a fracture within the next 10 years. Unlike the BMD, which simply measures bone quantity, FRAX could be characterized as measuring overall bone quality. By taking into account a dozen factors related to bone health, it gives a fuller picture of future fracture risk than the BMD alone. Although BMD can be included as a factor in the FRAX, the latter can be used instead of BMD to assess fracture risk in regions where a BMD is difficult to obtain.

Treatment

Although circumstances such as severe trauma may cause a bone fracture in a person with healthy bone, a fracture is very often a signal that bone quality has deteriorated. There is a saying that "fracture leads to fracture," which is a kind of shorthand for the fact that the biggest risk of re-fracture is in the first year after a fracture has occurred. The risk remains quite high in the second year and after that declines at a relatively modest rate.

This imminent risk of re-fracture has real implications for treatment. In the past, an initial fracture was not necessarily seen as a warning sign that another fracture might be just around the corner. We now know, though, that a fracture indicates that a re-fracture may reasonably be anticipated. In most cases, an immediate assessment of bone health should be done after an initial fracture to determine whether it is time to begin treatment for osteoporosis. And if treatment is required, there are choices about which is appropriate.

In general, there are two categories of drug therapy for osteoporosis: *antiresorptive medications* that slow bone erosion, thereby tipping the scale in favour of the bone-building cells, and *bone-formulating medications* that strengthen existing bone while also adding new bone. Most currently available osteoporosis drug therapies in Canada are in the antiresorptive category.

Antiresorptive medications

Most antiresorptive drugs are bisphosphonates. They work by preventing the activity of the osteoclast cells and thereby slowing down bone erosion. There are currently four bisphosphonates for the prevention and treatment of osteoporosis in postmenopausal women and men approved by Health Canada and available by prescription in Canada:

- Etidronate was approved in 1995 to prevent and treat osteoporosis. It is taken for 2 weeks followed by 2 ½ months of calcium supplementation. This cycle is repeated every 3 months.
- Alendronate was approved in 1996 to prevent and treat osteoporosis. It is taken once weekly, with a glass of water, before eating. Individuals are instructed to remain upright and not to eat or drink for at least 30 minutes. The problem with some of the generic versions is that the coating of the tablets may dissolve in the esophagus and cause local

irritation and poor absorption of the drug when compared with the branded tablet, which dissolves further down in the gastro-intestinal tract.

- Risedronate was approved in 2000 to prevent and treat osteoporosis. It is taken weekly or monthly (depending on dosage), with a glass of water first thing in the morning, on an empty stomach, at least 30 minutes before consuming the first food, drink (other than plain water), and/or any other medication of the day. Patients should not lie down for at least 30 minutes after taking the medication.
- Zoledronic acid was approved by Health Canada in 2007 for the treatment of osteoporosis in postmenopausal women. This medication is purchased by the patient and then administered by a health care professional intravenously for 15 minutes once a year.

Side effects from using bisphosphonates are minimal but can include gastro-intestinal symptoms such as nausea and abdominal pain, altered bowel habit, rashes, and temporary alterations in taste. As with any drug, there are also extremely rare, potentially serious side effects, so you should consult your physician with any concerns. A majority of patients discontinue these therapies because of the side effects. Generally, there is little benefit being on these drugs for more than five to seven years, so talk with your doctor if you need to review your status.

Another drug called denosumab is a newer, more precise antiresorptive therapy: it affects both the bone-building cells and the bone-eroding cells and tips activity towards the osteoblasts, effectively deactivating the osteoclasts. Denosumab is delivered with a single injection every six months, so after one shot, patients are done for half a year. Nothing to remember also means nothing to forget. There is now 10 years of research that shows not only improvement in bone density with denosumab but also improvement in fracture rates, a marker for bone quality. Significantly, the 10-year data involve people who were 10 years younger when they started taking denosumab—in other words, the research shows that their bone health actually *improved* as they aged! This is a remarkable development because age itself is a risk factor for osteoporosis. It is also extremely reassuring, as we know the whole story of bone health involves ongoing fracture reduction.

Bone-formulating medications

As I mentioned above, most of the osteoporosis drugs in Canada are antiresorptives, but some effective bone-formulating drugs are now available here as well. Side effects of these drugs are relatively rare because they target specific cellular mechanisms; however, as with any prescription, you should discuss the entire treatment protocol with your doctor.

Synthetic parathyroid hormone, which is available in a drug called teriparatide, activates the bone-building part of the bone remodelling cycle. It appears to activate bone remodelling by acting directly on osteoblast activity so that new bone is generated and added to the skeleton faster than old bone is broken down.

Teriparatide is used to treat postmenopausal women and men with severe osteoporosis who are at high risk of further fracture. Ideally the patient will not have been on previous bisphosphonate therapy, but the medication is approved for those who have failed on or who have been unable to tolerate previous osteoporosis therapy. It is taken as a daily injection into the thigh or abdominal wall for a maximum of 24 months. We know that bone loss can easily recur, so many patients may then go on to a second medication to help maintain the bone formation achieved.

And finally, Health Canada recently approved a drug that is an entirely new approach to treatment of osteoporosis and fracture risk. Greater understanding of bone biology indicates that there is a signalling pathway that regulates bone formation and resorption. The new drug, romosozumab, is a humanized monoclonal antibody that binds to the protein sclerostin. Sclerostin's normal role is to inhibit the signalling pathway for bone formation, but this function is prevented when romosozumab binds to sclerostin. In effect, romosozumab blocks sclerostin and allows the signalling pathway to become activated. A number of studies have shown that use of romosozumab leads to rapid bone formation and bone density gains.

Treatment involves two injections under the skin, one after the other, once a month for 12 months. Studies have shown an 18 percent gain in bone in that year. Once this powerful drug has increased bone density, patients can go on one of the antiresorptive drugs to maintain the bone that has been built. A major study of romosozumab showed there was also a 75 percent reduction of fracture risk in that first year, and that the 75 percent reduction of risk was maintained in the second year among the same patients who had begun denosumab treatment. Romosozumab acts as a foundation drug to build back bone, with an antiresorptive drug stabilizing the gains.

The discussion of romosozumab among osteoporosis professionals includes the question of what to do now: do we wait and use this drug only for people who have experienced severe bone loss, or do we also use it for people who are just beginning to lose bone? While that debate continues, and whatever the conclusion, let's keep in mind that we now have several effective treatments for osteoporosis. And beyond that, research into newer and better treatments is ongoing.

Bottom Line on Bones

Let's recap. Osteoporosis is a disease that can profoundly affect a person's quality of life as the result of painful and serious fractures. Age, previous fractures, and a family history of osteoporosis are risk factors. A healthy diet that provides adequate calcium, vitamin D, regular exercise, and appropriate screening can help prevent osteoporosis. And drug treatments for osteoporosis are available to slow down bone erosion or speed up bone formation.

Exercise is, of course, an important component of bone health and is vital at every age. Exercise will improve your bone health; it keeps your posture aligned and bones strong, especially if you do weight-bearing exercises that force you to work against gravity, such as walking, jogging, hiking, climbing stairs, and dancing.

Exercise also helps build muscle strength, which can help prevent falls and thereby avoid fractures. And there's a bonus: people who exercise regularly have lower rates of dementia, heart disease, cancer, diabetes, and many other chronic diseases.

So, this may not be a sexy, "hot-off-the press" topic that has been top of mind for you, but avoidance of osteoporosis (if possible) and treatment of osteoporosis (if avoidance is not possible) are extremely important in healthy aging, healthy living, and ongoing independence. This is an issue that deserves your time and attention now ... before you become one of those fracture statistics!

No bones about it—bone health supports healthy aging!

8

INTIMATE DIFFERENCES

Sexuality and Health

*L*et's talk about sex, baby. Let's talk about you and me. Thank you to Salt-N-Pepa for those inspiring words! Unlike the people in the pop song, though, in this case the "you" is you, and the "me" is your doctor. So yes, let's talk about sex, about sexual function, about what is considered normal and expected, and about what may perhaps be unexpected.

Your sexual health matters. Every woman deserves the opportunity to discuss her medical issues—including any sexual health issues—with her primary care provider. That conversation, however, often just does not happen. A study called the CLOSER study, which looked at the impact of the genitourinary syndrome of menopause (GSM), reviewed many sexual issues, including the comfort of both doctors and patients in talking about genital/sexual issues. Most patients were open to talking to their doctors if they were asked, but most were never specifically asked about their sexual health. Apparently, doctors felt their patient would bring up any sexual health issues; similarly, patients, who often felt constrained, believed their doctor would initiate discussion of sexual health if it were important.

And it is reasonable—in fact, desirable—for your primary care provider to ask you screening questions about your sexual health when you are having a general checkup or review of your health. I was honoured to be part of the writing group that developed a guide for doctors to help them identify sexual concerns and problems in women. A globally renowned organization of experts on women's sexual health, the International Society for the Study of Women's Sexual Health (ISSWSH), published this report in the Mayo Clinic Proceedings in 2019.

The first question we recommended a doctor ask is simple: "Are you currently involved in a relationship?" or "Are you sexually active?" If the answer is yes, the next question is, "Do you have any concerns?" Maybe yes and maybe no. On the other hand, if the answer to the question about sexual activity is no, the next question is, "Do you have any concerns that you would like to discuss or that may have contributed to the lack of sexual behaviour?" Such questions help to legitimize the importance of assessing sexual function and normalizing this issue as part of the usual health history and physical examination.

A satisfying sexual life is part of the normal expectations of good health. What is normal, though, may differ from person to person. Sexual desire and sexual response involve many aspects of our lives and are complex areas to understand. The intersection of biology, psychology, socio-cultural norms, and interpersonal relationships all impact how we feel and how we perceive ourselves and our partners, and that in turn affects our sexual expression.

Biology is basic to our sexuality, encompassing our physical health and including the endocrine system, which regulates the release of hormones into the bloodstream. Psychology is important, too—mood changes, depression or anxiety, and impairment of self-image as we age can all affect our sexual health. Socio-cultural norms and the specifics of our upbringing affect us as well because they set up expectations about what a healthy sex life should look like. And one can hardly talk about healthy sexuality without considering interpersonal relationships, both current and previous, because they have a lasting influence on our experience. Interpersonal relationships often inform how we deal with life stressors—the health, well-being, and support of partners plays a big part in that and can have a major impact on our sexual satisfaction.

So, what exactly makes for healthy sexual functioning? To begin with, it is important to clarify that there is no one right answer. What is right for one person or couple is not necessarily right for another. As a physician, I think one of the most important questions I can ask about a patient's sexual health is: "Are you distressed by the current state of your sex life?" Whether you have sex easily and often or rarely and with difficulty, if you and your partner are on the same wavelength and not distressed, then we can move on and discuss other health issues. There is no need to medicalize sexual function if neither you nor your partner is distressed by your current situation, whatever it may be.

However, there are a great number of women who are distressed, and their distress can show remarkable similarities. So much so, in fact, that ISSWSH identifies a broad spectrum of sexual complaints and categorizes them into specific disorders. The ISSWSH has been very active in distinguishing between various disorders and in helping to contextualize issues and make them more understandable, both to the women who experience them and to their doctors.

According to Dr. Sheryl Kingsberg, past president of the North American Menopause Society (NAMS) and author of a recent textbook on sexual health for women, the loss of desire can affect how women see themselves. They are more likely to experience negative impacts on self-esteem, body image, and self-confidence, and they often feel isolated, ashamed, and inadequate. They may reject any intimacy, such as hugging or kissing, since they do not want to encourage an expectation of sex. Partners may feel rejected and lonely.

If your current situation is distressing, then let's figure out why and how to make things more positive. There are a number of issues that may be affecting your sexual function. For instance, a quite common problem is a medical issue, such as an operation, injury, depression, and other disease. Or you may be on medications that affect sexual desire and/or response, and alcohol can certainly have a bearing. Pregnancy, recent childbirth, and menopausal hormonal changes can all impact function. Perhaps you experience pain with intercourse or have complex regional pain syndrome. You may be very stressed and/or fatigued. Your partner may have personal issues, a serious illness, or other concerns that affect you both. And finally, perhaps your relationship itself is an issue.

Factors such as these can affect your desire, your interest, and your ability to feel satisfied in your sex life. These are primary issues in impaired sexual function and need to be dealt with. Whether it is changing medication or recovering from surgery or seeking marital counselling, improvement in sexual function depends on the resolution of the primary problem.

EVALUATION

You may feel there is a problem, but how do you get a handle on it? One way is to use a simple assessment tool called the Decreased Sexual Desire Screener (DSDS). To complete it, let's first assume that you are not experiencing any of the issues mentioned above. Then answer the following four questions:

1.   In the past, was your level of sexual desire or interest good and satisfying to you?

2.   Has there been a decrease in your level of sexual desire or interest?

3.   Are you bothered by your decreased level of sexual desire or interest?

4.   Would you like your level of sexual desire or interest to increase?

If you answer yes to each of these questions and you don't have any of the major issues just discussed, then you would qualify for the diagnosis of generalized hypoactive sexual desire disorder (HSDD), a relatively new concept in women's sexual health and one of several female sexual dysfunctions recognized by ISSWSH.

Why is it important to know this? Well, firstly, because it lets you know that you are not alone. It is estimated that 10 percent of the female population suffers from HSDD. When I talk to women about their sexual distress, they often say, "I thought it was just me!" Most find it reassuring to learn that many other women are having the same type of experience.

Women who experience HSDD have a variety of complaints. Among them is reduced spontaneous desire, that is, a lack of sexual thoughts or fantasies. And there may be reduced or absent responsive desire to erotic cues or stimulation. There is a loss of desire to either initiate or participate in sexual activity, often leading to avoidance behaviours such as dodging hugs or kisses from a partner, as mentioned above. Result: personal distress, frustration, sadness, loss, or worry … and a partner who often feels rejected and diminished, and so withdraws.

Distress may be a psychological state, but it often has physiological underpinnings, so let's take a look at the physiology of sexual function and its psychological effects. Many physiological systems depend upon the interplay of two opposing mechanisms, an interplay that helps to keep the entire organism—the human being—in balance. In bone, for example, it is the interplay of bone-building cells and bone-resorbing cells. In sexual function, it is the interplay of excitation and inhibition.

Physiological exciters include certain hormones linked to pleasure, such as dopamine, norepinephrine, estrogen, testosterone, and nitric oxide. These hormones stimulate various parts of the brain, creating a faster, easier, and generally greater response to sexual stimuli. Psychosocial and cultural factors such as feelings of love, attraction to a partner, fantasy, and courtship can also be stimulating. All play a role in excitation.

On the other hand, chemical inhibitors of sexual function include serotonin, prolactin, endocannabinoids, and opioids. Psychosocial factors such as negative thoughts and emotions, stress and anger, and partner issues all have potentially dampening effects that can lead to sexual avoidance and negativity.

The result is, at best, a slower and more difficult response to sexual stimuli; at worst, no response at all.

There is some interesting research that studies activation of different areas of the brain in women who experience HSDD and women who exhibit healthy sexual functioning. This research shows physical differences in the way women in the two groups respond when viewing erotic videos, sports videos, and relaxing images. Functional magnetic resonance imaging (fMRI) scans indicate that the areas of the brain activated in women without pathology were not activated in women with HSDD. Furthermore, given the interplay of exciters and inhibitors, it seems almost intuitive that as certain areas of the brain begin to react to sexual stimuli, other areas of the brain need to shut down. In other words, the left side of the brain needs to stop multi-tasking so that we can relax and focus on pleasure! These studies reveal that no such shutdown occurred in women with HSDD.

TREATMENT

Let's assume you are distressed by a lack of sexual interest and response that is due to HSDD and you want to change the situation. What can you do?

Well, I am almost always thinking about personalized medicine, and that means tailoring the treatment options to the individual. When I take your history and review the issues with you, there may be several treatment options that suit the problem, but not all of them are likely to suit you. In sexual health, it is not a one-size-fits-all situation (honestly, I don't know when it ever is!). So, let's partner together, look at the treatment options, and then decide where to begin.

The first intervention is education, for both you and your partner. It is important to understand what modifiable factors known to inhibit sexual function are at play in a given individual. It is also important to understand the range of choices of treatment—from the very basic to the newer and more sophisticated approaches—and we need to understand changes in normal sexual function that come with aging.

Some women respond well to different types of therapy. Psychotherapy, cognitive behavioural therapy (CBT), mindfulness-based CBT, sex therapy, and couples' therapy can all be of benefit. Some prefer one-on-one therapy while others respond better with group therapy.

Mindfulness meditation, for example, with its emphasis on nonjudgmental awareness and its goal of being always in the present moment, is often helpful in alleviating cognitive distraction during sexual activity: it teaches women how to focus on a particular sensation and not get distracted by ongoing stresses and anxieties. Mindfulness has been used for people with chronic pain, anxiety, and depression. In sexual therapy, an eight-week group mindfulness program was shown to improve sexual desire and overall function and decrease sex-related distress. That seems to be a good start, a step in the right direction, and for some women such an intervention alone may be sufficient.

For other women, though, issues persist despite their best efforts. Even when external forces are all aligned, when a woman has good rapport with an intimate partner, when she feels positive about herself, when she is taking no medications that are known to suppress sexual function, and when she has no major illnesses or depression, still she may lose interest in or cease to enjoy sexual activity. For such a woman, psychotherapy does not seem to be the solution.

However, there may be a pharmaceutical solution. In fact, there are two new drugs available in North America for the treatment of HSDD. As mentioned, it is estimated that HSDD affects one in every ten adult women. The pharmacotherapies being investigated include hormone therapies and agents that affect the central nervous system (CNS), specifically to increase sexual excitation or decrease sexual inhibition.

While doctors have prescribed hormones, including testosterone, for various conditions, there is no approved testosterone product in North America for use in women. Some physicians will prescribe it off label for HSDD, which means it is not being used for the usual and approved reasons. However, as discussed by the NAMS, the research is mixed as to its effectiveness in treating this condition.

Bupropion is a CNS medication used for anxiety and for smoking cessation. It blocks the reuptake of dopamine and norepinephrine, leading to these neurotransmitters being present in the brain for a longer time. Theoretically, this would increase excitation. Because it was approved to treat other conditions, use of bupropion for sexual dysfunction would have to be considered off label; it has not yet been studied as a treatment for HSDD.

However, a drug called flibanserin has been studied and is now available in both Canada and United States. Initially developed as a possible treatment for depression, it was found to increase the excitatory pathways and to inhibit the ability of serotonin to activate the inhibitory pathways. In other words, in terms of sexual function, its action is like stepping on the gas and not allowing your foot to hit the brake. Flibanserin was found to have a positive effect on women with HSDD.

How was that effect measured? Very importantly, it was measured by the women in the study themselves, in that they reported increased desire, decreased distress, and an increase is what they considered to be sexually satisfying events. This was not measured in number of orgasms or frequency of sex but rather in the women's reports of positive sexual experience.

Another therapy, now available in the United States but not yet in Canada, is bremelanotide. This is a CNS medication that is injected when needed by the patient. It targets melanocortin receptors in the brain that appear to be involved in cognition and mood regulation.

Other medications are being studied as treatments for HSDD; in general, they are all CNS drugs, affecting the delicate balance between excitation and inhibition. We know that the erectile dysfunction medications for men are all about vasodilation and blood flow, but for most women with HSDD, drugs that act on the central nervous system appear most effective in the balance and the overall integration of various physiological and psychological factors.

No matter where you find yourself on the sexual satisfaction continuum—highly satisfied, deeply dissatisfied, or somewhere in the middle—it is important to realize that sexual health is a normal component of health. It is not frivolous or self-indulgent to think about your sexuality, to assess your level of satisfaction, and to discuss any concerns with your doctor. We are all entitled to understand our experience of intimacy, or lack of intimacy, and how it affects our overall health.

Afterword

I'd like to conclude this book with a final reminder: to a significant extent your health is up to you. No, I have not forgotten the fact that sometimes health problems occur due to non-modifiable risks such as genetics and family history, environmental factors, age, ethnicity, and gender. But the message I hope you take from this book is that by making wise lifestyle choices—including good nutrition, regular physical activity, effective sleep hygiene, social engagement, avoidance of smoking, and moderate alcohol consumption—you can exert significant control over important modifiable risk factors such as your blood pressure, your cholesterol levels, your weight, and the level of stress in your life.

I sincerely hope you will make the decision to take your health into your own hands and make it a priority every day.

Staying strong, healthy, and connected can extend the period of your life in which you remain vital and independent. It can improve your day-to-day experience of life through better outlook, better posture, better balance, better decision making. And it will make you better able to cope with any chronic disorder or illness that may appear in your later years.

This book is not a guarantee—though I wish it could be! Rather it is a guide to point you to the choices you can make for a long and healthy life. The recommendations included in it are all based on recent health research. But keep in mind that scientific inquiry into human health is advancing at a remarkable pace, and as a result of new discoveries and new understandings health recommendations change. Try to keep on top of major changes—reading the health section of your daily newspaper is one way to do this. Or check out your favourite health-related websites from time to time. Staying well informed could be considered another wise lifestyle choice.

I mentioned earlier that life is a journey, full of adventures, challenges, victories, and temporary defeats. I wish you safe travels, and I hope this book will be a useful guide to you on your journey.

Appendix

A. NUTRITION
B. EXERCISE
C. VIRTUAL MEDICAL APPOINTMENT

I discuss nutrition in Chapter 1 and exercise in Chapter 2. This appendix includes some important additional information that relates to nutrition (Section A) and to exercise (Section B) but that does not fit well into the chapters themselves. It also includes a ten-step guide to help you prepare for and get the most benefit from a virtual medical appointment (Section C).

A. NUTRITION
Body Mass Index
As mentioned in Chapter 1, Body Mass Index (BMI) is a measure of body fat based on height and weight. It is a useful tool for determining whether a person's weight is proportionate

to their height. In other words, are they underweight, normal weight, overweight, or obese?

It is a useful tool but not a foolproof tool. For instance, it is not used for

- children who have not yet finished growing or for the elderly, because it would often indicate that they are underweight when in fact their weight may be healthy for their age
- women who are pregnant or lactating, because the BMI calculation cannot reflect the normal changes in their body composition
- people who have a high proportion of lean muscle mass, such as weight trainers and athletes, because they may have a higher BMI but not be at greater risk of developing health problems as muscle weighs more than fat

Table 1 shows the Health Canada Health Risk Classification According to Body Mass Index (BMI).

How to calculate Body Mass Index

Body Mass Index is a simple calculation using a person's height and weight. The formula is BMI $= kg/m^2$ where kg is a person's weight in kilograms and m^2 is their height in

Table 1: Health Canada Health Risk Classification
According to Body Mass Index (BMI)

Classification	BMI Category (kg/m²)	Risk of developing health problems
Underweight	< 18.5	Increased
Normal weight	18.5 – 24.9	Least
Overweight	25.0 – 29.9	Increased
Obese Class 1	30.0 – 34.9	High
Obese Class 2	35.0 – 39.9	Very High
Obese Class 3	> = 40.0	Extremely High

Notes: For persons 65 years and older the "normal" range may begin slightly above BMI 18.5 and extend into the "overweight" range. **To clarify risk for each individual, other factors such as lifestyle habits, fitness level, and presence or absence of other health risk conditions also need to be considered.**

Source: Health Canada. Canadian Guidelines for Body Weight Classification in Adults. Ottawa: Minister of Public Works and Government Services Canada; 2003. (www.hc-sc.gc.ca/fn-an/nutrition/weights-poids/guide-ld-adult/bmi_chart-graph_imc-eng.php) [Health Canada BMI; Archived June 24, 2013.]

metres squared. A BMI of 25.0 or more is overweight, while the healthy range is 18.5 to 24.9. BMI applies to most adults 18 to 65 years. You can find an online BMI calculator on the website of the Canadian Diabetes Association at **www.diabetes.ca/managing-my-diabetes/tools---resources/body-mass-index-(bmi)-calculator.**

The MIND diet

The MIND diet is a hybrid of the Mediterranean diet and the DASH diet. MIND, of course, is also an acronym; it stands for Mediterranean-DASH Intervention for Neurodegenerative Delay. It is based on years' worth of research about the foods and nutrients that have good—and bad—effects on the functioning of the brain over time.

This relatively new diet could significantly lower a person's risk of developing Alzheimer's disease, even if it is not meticulously followed. So say the developers of the diet—nutritional epidemiologist Martha Clare Morris and her colleagues at Rush University Medical Center in Chicago—in a paper published in the online journal *Alzheimer's & Dementia: The Journal of the Alzheimer's Association.*

Their study showed that the MIND diet lowered the risk of Alzheimer's by as much as 53 percent in participants who adhered to the diet rigorously and by about 35 percent in those who followed it moderately well. The researchers got interesting results when they compared the MIND with the Mediterranean and the DASH diets. These diets were also found to reduce the incidence of Alzheimer's when followed meticulously—54 percent and 39 percent, respectively—but the benefit from moderate adherence to either of them was negligible. Yes, it takes meticulous adherence to get the greatest benefit, but the good news is that the MIND diet is easier to follow.

The MIND diet identifies 15 dietary components: 10 "brain healthy" food groups and five unhealthy food groups. Unlike many diets, the MIND regime is not highly prescribed—you don't have to count calories, you don't have to eat certain foods on certain days or at a certain time of the day—and that makes it easier to follow. Here is how it works.

You eat things from the 10 brain-healthy food groups:

- Green leafy vegetables (like spinach and salad greens): At least six servings a week
- Other vegetables: At least one a day
- Nuts: Five servings a week
- Berries: Two or more servings a week
- Beans: At least three servings a week
- Whole grains: Three or more servings a day
- Fish: Once a week
- Poultry (like chicken or turkey): Two times a week
- Olive oil: Use it as your main cooking oil
- Wine: One glass a day

And you avoid foods from the five unhealthy food groups:

- Red meat: Less than four servings a week
- Butter and margarine: Less than a tablespoon daily
- Cheese: Less than one serving a week
- Pastries and sweets: Less than five servings a week
- Fried or fast food: Less than one serving a week

The MIND diet gives you a lot of leeway to eat the things you like when you want to eat them. For many, it becomes more an aspect of a healthy lifestyle and less an onerous dietary regime. And there is even more good news: the MIND diet also has beneficial effects on heart health.

Online resources for other nutritional information

- For information about the Mediterranean diet: **www.mayoclinic.org/healthy-lifestyle/ nutrition-and-healthy-eating/in-depth/ mediterranean-diet/art-20047801**
- For information about the DASH diet: **www.nhlbi.nih.gov/health/health-topics /topics/dash-eating-plan**
- For an illustrated explanation of Canada's Food Guide: **www.food=guide.canada.ca/ en/?wbdisabled=true**

Cholesterol

What should my cholesterol level be?

Your doctor will measure your cholesterol level. If the total level is high, a second test may be done to measure the levels of HDL and LDL.

If your total level is high because of a high LDL level, you may be at higher risk of heart disease or stroke. If your total level is high only because of a high HDL level, you're not at higher risk.

Target LDL, HDL, and total cholesterol: HDL levels

Your doctor can determine your target levels based on your risk factors for heart disease, using your age, gender, total and HDL cholesterol, blood pressure level, medications, and smoking status. Note that recommendations regarding optimal cholesterol levels change as more research is conducted, but the rule of thumb seems to be that lower is better.

- An LDL cholesterol level of less than 3.0 mmol/L is best.
- An HDL above 1.0 mmol/L is best.
- If your risk is low, your LDL cholesterol should be less than 5.0 mmol/L and total cholesterol HDL-C ratio should be less than 6.0.
- If your risk is moderate, your LDL cholesterol should be less than 3.5 mmol/ and total cholesterol HDL-C ratio should be less than 5.
- If your risk is high, your LDL cholesterol should be less than 1.8 mmol/L and total cholesterol HDL-C ratio should be less than 4.0.
- An HDL cholesterol level of less than 1.0 mmol/L means you're at higher risk for heart disease.
- If you have diabetes, your LDL should be less than 1.8 mmol/L.
- If you've already had a heart attack your LDL needs to be less than 1.8 mmol/L.

For advice on how to manage your cholesterol levels, see: **www.heartandstroke.ca/heart-disease/risk-and-prevention /condition-risk-factors/managing-cholesterol**.

Calcium content of various foods

In Chapter 1 (on nutrition) and again in Chapter 7 (on bone health), I discussed how important it is to make sure your diet includes adequate calcium. If you glance at the table of nutrition facts on a carton of milk or many other dairy products, it's easy to see how much calcium a serving contains. But what about all the other dietary sources of calcium? How can you tell how much calcium you're getting in a serving of broccoli, or kale, or grapefruit? Try the Osteoporosis Canada website—it's a great source of information. This URL will take you to a fairly comprehensive table that shows the calcium content of many common foods: **www.osteo-porosis.ca/bone-health-osteoporosis/nutrition/calcium -requirements/**.

B. EXERCISE

The official **Canadian Physical Activity Guidelines** are developed and published by the **Canadian Society for Exercise Physiology** (CSEP). You can find guidelines for early childhood (ages 0–4 years), childhood (ages 5–17 years), adulthood (ages 18–64 years), and late adulthood (65 years and older) at **www.csep.ca**. CSEP also publishes activity guidelines for special populations—people with multiple sclerosis, spinal cord injury, and Parkinson's disease.

The **Heart and Stroke Foundation of Canada** offers exercise recommendations for children, adults, and seniors. You can check them out at **www.heartandstroke.ca/healthy-living /stay-active/how-much-physical-activity-do-you-need**.

In addition, **Osteoporosis Canada** publishes exercise guidelines for people with osteoporosis. Information on the types of exercises they recommend, including strength training, posture training, balance training, and weight-bearing aerobic activity can be found on their website at **www.osteoporosis.ca/bone-health-osteoporosis/exercises -for-healthy-bones/**. If you have osteoporosis, be sure to consult with your doctor before you begin an exercise program.

C. TEN STEPS OF A VIRTUAL MEDICAL APPOINTMENT

As I mentioned in the preface, the importance of social distancing during the COVID-19 pandemic has resulted in many medical visits being done virtually, either online or by phone.

This method of patient care, already in fairly limited use before the pandemic, has become more broadly used since. It has been found to be quite appropriate for a wide variety of medical issues. Going forward, in all likelihood, it will evolve into a regular part of medical care, so here are a few basic steps to follow so that your virtual care visit is efficient, effective, and productive:

1. Book an appointment. Sounds simple, but remember that doctors are busy people and in an average day meet with many patients who have pressing questions and concerns. Booking an appointment time is the most efficient way to meet virtually: it gives both you and your doctor time to prepare—you, to organize your thoughts and concerns; and your doctor, to review your file and be ready to answer your questions.

2. Make sure you are comfortable with your computer, your e-mail, and your phone. Test your audio and video so you can see and hear clearly. Be sure you have downloaded the most appropriate browser in order to connect seamlessly on your device.

3. Have the priority reason for the call (and related main questions) ready to go to ensure it can be dealt with first in the time allotted. Organize any other, less urgent, questions and write them down in order of importance to make sure you use the time you have as efficiently as possible. Presumably there will not be an endless list of issues for you and your doctor to focus on; less pressing matters can likely wait and be dealt with in another visit.

4. Have all your medications handy when you make the call, if not in bottles beside you then in a list with the dosages and refill dates. This is really important since your doctor can't know what the "small white pill" is that you take. There are often generic medications, and the look of the generic pill may be vastly different from the look of the brand-name pill even though the drug is the same.

5. Have your current weight and blood pressure available. They are important starting points for this appointment.

6. Have your immunization record handy as it may be necessary to determine when you had your last tetanus shot—for example, if you are calling about a burn or a bite.

7. Be in a quiet place away from interruptions. It is hard to focus on a conversation when there is noise (like a barking dog or other distracting pet) or other disruptions during the call.

8. Be in a private place to ensure confidentiality. This makes it possible to discuss personal issues that you would be uncomfortable raising when others are around; you should not feel limited in what you say or how you say it. It also allows your doctor to ask personal questions that they would not ask you in front of others.

9. If you need assistance, perhaps due to poor hearing or poor vision, plan your call when your partner or a friend can be there to help you. (If you have a sensitive, personal issue to discuss, this may mean that an office visit is more appropriate.)

10. Finally, just as with an office visit, a virtual visit involves informed consent, so you can rest assured that it is a confidential visit and that there will be a record of it in your medical chart.

Acknowledgements

T here are many people I would like to thank for the inspiration and support they have provided—in my life and in the writing of this book.

First of all my family—my loving, giving, and endlessly supportive husband Shelley; my daughter Ashley, who bought me a Fitbit, cheers me on every day and teaches me about true bravery; my son Jared and his wife Yael, incredible role models for me to emulate—all of whom have been there for me every step of the way. Thanks as well to my special grandchildren, Ethan and Ryder, Elielle and Raphael, who remind me of the joy and wonder of life itself.

I am grateful to my extended family, for I am truly blessed with my fabulous brother Eric and his incredible wife Sharon, my courageous sister Carren, my nieces and nephews and their spouses and children, my cousins, my in-laws and out-laws. I am forever indebted to my late uncle, Dr. Marvin Lipton, my mentor, both personally and professionally, who set the highest standard with ease and grace, and encouraged me every step of the way. I have learned so much from my husband's family, especially from my 99-year-old mother-in-law, Doris. They are all a gift without measure.

Dr. Marla Shapiro, for her constant support in our medical journey together—we have been friends and colleagues since our medical school days, and she is abundantly generous with both her knowledge and mentorship.

Also my many other colleagues, too many to mention by name, with whom I have worked over the years. They have taught me many things and shared our busy days. No one does it alone. Medicine, indeed, is a team sport, and I have been lucky to have many wonderful people working with me on my team.

Susan Caldwell of Metrix Group, for her close reading of an early draft, for her insightful suggestions, and for her guidance and wisdom as a mentor and friend.

My editor, Tom Churchill, whose commitment was unwavering and whose guidance and expertise was invaluable as this book took shape.

Marjorie Wallens of MJW Communications, whose counsel has been instrumental and whose support was ongoing.

The special women in my life: Beverly, Liliane, Phyllis, and Andree, and many other good and true friends, who are always there for me, helping to share this journey.

The editors, designers, and all the other wonderful people at Barlow Books, who turned my manuscript into the volume you now hold.

And finally—and wholeheartedly—my patients, who have trusted me with their health care since I started my medical career decades ago. I have learned so much about how to practise medicine compassionately, empathetically, and effectively from each of you. It has been a joyful, emotional, sometimes very sad, but always special relationship, and I feel very lucky to have had you in my life.

There is an African saying that states, "If you want to go fast, go alone. If you want to go far, go together." Yes, indeed, we can and will go far together.

Notes

1 The Edible Feast: Diet and Nutrition

The obesity epidemic is a growing problem. The following article looks at the long-term trajectory of obesity rates and the potential consequences for life expectancy: Olshansky, SJ et al. A potential decline in life expectancy in the United States in the 21st century. *New England Journal of Medicine.* 352:1138–1145, 2005.

World Health Organization. Obesity and Overweight. Fact sheet no. 3011. Available at **www.who.int/news-room/fact-sheets.** Accessed October 5, 2013.

The percentage of Canadian men and women who are obese or overweight is from Statistics Canada: **www150.statcan. gc.ca/t1/tbl1/en/tv.action?pid=1310037301**.

Information on the relationship between waist circumference and obesity comes from WebMD: **www.webmd.com/diet/ guide/calculating-your-waist-circumference**.

Information on the negative health outcomes for a person eating a 2,000-calorie-per-day diet and ingesting just 22 grams of saturated fat or less per day comes from the Cleveland Clinic: **https://my.clevelandclinic.org/health /articles/11208-fat-what-you-need-to-know**.

The positive effects of HDL cholesterol are discussed at **www.webmd.com/cholesterol-management/guide/hdl-cholesterol-the-good-cholesterol**.

2   Pump It Up and Let It Rest: Exercise and Sleep

Much of the information in this chapter about the benefits of regular exercise is based on publications of the Heart and Stroke Foundation of Canada (**www.heartandstroke.com**) and the Canadian Society for Exercise Physiology (**www.csep. ca/home**).

Personal experience led Arianna Huffington to research the effects of sleep deprivation, some of which are discussed in this chapter. Her book, *The Sleep Revolution: Transforming Your Life, One Night at a Time* (New York: Penguin Random House, 2016), presents the conclusions of that research as well as strategies for getting better, more restorative sleep.

3   Healthy Hemispheres: The Aging Brain

The long quotation about gender differences in brain structure on the first page of this chapter is from a Columbia University article, *Male vs. Female: The Brain Differences*. It can be accessed at **www.columbia.edu/itc/anthropology/v1007/ jakabovics/mf2.html**.

Women's Brain Health Initiative has played an enormous role in ensuring that research into brain health in Canada is applicable to women as well as men. I encourage you to visit their website at **womensbrainhealth.org** for up-to-date information on the organization and on some of the current research findings that have informed this chapter.

The Alzheimer Society of Canada is an invaluable source of information about Alzheimer's disease and other dementias—you will find everything from recognizing the signs of dementia, understanding what dementia is, living with dementia, and the latest research findings on their website: **www.alzheimer.ca**.

The graphic on blood flow to the hippocampus before and after exercise comes from the following study: Cotman, CW et al. Exercise: a behavioral intervention to enhance brain health and plasticity. *Trends in Neurosciences.* 25(6):295–301, 2002.

The two following studies also provide information on the effects of exercise on the brain:

- Ravaglia, G et al. Physical activity and dementia risk in the elderly. *Neurology.* 6(70):1786–1794, May 6, 2008. Published online December 19, 2007.
- Verdelho, A et al. Physical activity prevents progression for cognitive impairment and vascular dementia: results from the LADIS (Leukoaraiosis and Disability) study. *Stroke.* 43(12):3331–3335, December 2012.

The surprising findings about how much impact meditation can have on brain physiology in just eight weeks comes from the following study: Hölze, Britta K et al. Mindfulness practice leads to increases in regional brain gray matter density. *Psychiatry Research: Neuroimaging.* 191(1):36–43, January 30, 2011.

The UCLA study about the link between meditation and increased brain volumes is Luders, E et al. The underlying anatomical correlates of long-term meditation: Larger hippo-campal and frontal volumes of gray matter. *Neuroimage*. 45(3): 672–678, April 15, 2009.

Other studies that are helpful in understanding the effects of meditation on the brain include these:

- Epel, E et al. Can meditation slow rate of cellular aging? Cognitive stress, mindfulness, and telomeres. *Annals of the New York Academy of Sciences*, 1172(1):34-53, 2009.
- Luders, E et al. Enhanced brain connectivity in long-term meditation practitioners. *Neuroimage*, 57(4):1308–1316, 2011.

The study about the effects of the Mediterranean diet on brain volume was led by Dr. Yian Gu, a researcher at Columbia University: Gu, Y et al. Mediterranean diet and brain structure in a multiethnic elderly cohort. *Neurology*. 85(20):1744–1751, November 17, 2015.

The fascinating information about the MIND diet being protective against Alzheimer's disease is found in the paper "MIND diet associated with reduced risk of Alzheimer's disease" by epidemiologist Martha Clare Morris and her colleagues at Rush University Medical Center in Chicago. It was published in *Alzheimer's & Dementia: The Journal of the Alzheimer's Association*. 11(9):1007–1014, September 2015. It was published online February 11, 2015.

The link between sleep problems and declining brain volume was first discovered through a remarkable study in the United Kingdom: Sexton, C et al. Poor sleep quality is associated with increased cortical atrophy in community-dwelling adults. *Neurology*. 83(11):967–973, September 9, 2014.

For background on the MoCA test, see Nasreddine, ZS et al. The Montreal Cognitive Assessment, MoCA: a brief screening tool for mild cognitive impairment. *Journal of the American Geriatric Society*. 53(4):695–699, April 2005.

4   The Value of Vaccines: Immunization-Preventable Diseases

The Canadian immunization guidelines in this chapter are based on recommendations of the National Advisory Committee on Immunization (NACI), which includes experts in the fields of pediatrics, infectious diseases, immunology, medical microbiology, internal medicine, and public health. NACI recommendations are then provided to Public Health Canada, the agency that gives us our national recommendations on immunization. Implementation of these recommendations is under provincial recommendations, which, unfortunately, leaves us with a patchwork of immunization schedules and uneven funding across the country.

The NACI makes it easy for doctors to access information on immunization by consulting the online resource called the

CIG, or Canadian Immunization Guide. The NACI website is **www.phac-aspc.gc.ca/naci-ccni**.

Information on immunization is also available for the public from Public Health Canada through Immunize Canada at **www.immunize.ca**.

5 Marking Middle Age: Menopause and After

The North American Menopause Society (NAMS) is a reliable source of up-to-date information on all aspects of menopause. I am certified by the society as a menopause practitioner and follow their guidelines in my practice. The information in this chapter is in line with these guidelines and with current research published by the society. For further information, please consult their website: **www.menopause.org**. NAMS and the Canadian Menopause Society, SIGMA, are both affiliated with the International Menopause Society.

The discussion of sexual response in menopausal and/or postmenopausal women is based on the research of Rosemary Basson, especially the following:

- Basson, R. Using a different model for female sexual response to address women's problematic low sexual desire. *Journal of Sex and Marital Therapy*, 2001; 27(5): 395–403.
- Basson, R. Hormones and sexuality: current complexities and future directions. *Maturitas*, 2007; 57(1):66–70.

The quotation about hormone therapy initiation and breast cancer mortality is from Mikkola, TS et al. Reduced risk of breast cancer mortality in women using postmenopausal hormone therapy: a Finnish nationwide comparative study. *Menopause*, July 25, 2016. Published online ahead of print.

6   Happy Valentine's Day:
Maintaining Heart Health

The Heart and Stroke Foundation of Canada (www.heartand-stroke.com) is a trusted source of information about heart health, and much of the information in this chapter is based on their research and recommendations.

Another excellent source of information about how to maintain a healthy heart is the book by Dr. Beth Abramson, *Heart Health for Canadians: The Definitive Guide* (Toronto: HarperCollins Canada, 2013).

7   Robust or Brittle?
Bone Health and Osteoporosis

Osteoporosis Canada is a reliable source of up-to-date information on all aspects of osteoporosis. Much of the content in this chapter, including information on the relationship between menopause and development of osteoporosis, is based on information from Osteoporosis Canada and is in line with guidelines of Osteoporosis Canada. For further information, please consult their website: **www.osteoporosis.ca**.

8   Intimate Differences: Sexuality and Health

If you would like to read further on issues in the medical approach to women's sexual health, please refer to the Mayo Clinic's Publication of *The International Society for the Study of Women's Sexual Health: Process of Care for the Identification of Sexual Concerns and Problems in Women.*

Appendix
Body Mass Index
For more information, see **www.canada.ca/en/health-canada/services/food-nutrition/healthy-eating/healthy-weights/canadian-guidelines-body-weight-classification-adults/body-mass-index-nomogram.html** [Health Canada BMI; Archived June 24, 2013] and Canadian Diabetes Association (**www.diabetes.ca**).

The MIND diet
For more information, see Rush University Medical Center **www.rush.edu/news/new-mind-diet-may-significantly**

-protect-against-alzheimers-disease WebMD: **www.webmd. com/alzheimers/features/mind-diet-alzheimers-disease#1.**

Cholesterol

For more information, see **www.heartandstroke.ca/heart -disease/risk-and-prevention/condition-risk-factors /managing-cholesterol.**

Index

About the Author

D r. Vivien Brown, a Toronto-based family physician, lectures around the world about healthy aging and women's health. She is past president of the Federation of Medical Women of Canada and vice president for North America for the Medical Women's International Association. In 2012, Brown was named Physician of the Year (Toronto region) by the Ontario College of Family Physicians. In 2018, she received the Media Award from the North American Menopause Society for her work in promoting women's health.

www.drvivienbrown.com
@DrVivienBrown

Notes

Notes